Casting Light on the Dark Side of Brain Imaging

Casting Light on the Dark Side of Brain Imaging

Edited by

Amir Raz

Institute for Interdisciplinary Brain and Behavioral Sciences, Chapman University, Irvine, California, United States

Department of Psychiatry, McGill University, Montreal, QC, Canada

Robert T. Thibault

Integrated Program in Neuroscience, McGill University, Montreal, QC, Canada

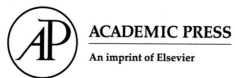

ACADEMIC PRESS

An imprint of Elsevier

Academic Press is an imprint of Elsevier
125 London Wall, London EC2Y 5AS, United Kingdom
525 B Street, Suite 1650, San Diego, CA 92101, United States
50 Hampshire Street, 5th Floor, Cambridge, MA 02139, United States
The Boulevard, Langford Lane, Kidlington, Oxford OX5 1GB, United Kingdom

Notices
Knowledge and best practice in this field are constantly changing. As new research and experience broaden our
understanding, changes in research methods, professional practices, or medical treatment may become
necessary.

Practitioners and researchers must always rely on their own experience and knowledge in evaluating and using
any information, methods, compounds, or experiments described herein. In using such information or methods
they should be mindful of their own safety and the safety of others, including parties for whom they have a
professional responsibility.

To the fullest extent of the law, neither the Publisher nor the authors, contributors, or editors, assume any
liability for any injury and/or damage to persons or property as a matter of products liability, negligence or
otherwise, or from any use or operation of any methods, products, instructions, or ideas contained in the
material herein.

British Library Cataloguing-in-Publication Data
A catalogue record for this book is available from the British Library

Library of Congress Cataloging-in-Publication Data
A catalog record for this book is available from the Library of Congress

ISBN: 978-0-12-816179-1

For Information on all Academic Press publications
visit our website at https://www.elsevier.com/books-and-journals

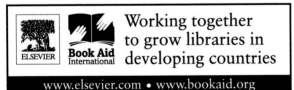

Working together
to grow libraries in
developing countries

www.elsevier.com • www.bookaid.org

Publisher: Nikki Levy
Acquisition Editor: Emily Ekle
Editorial Project Manager: Barbara Makinster
Production Project Manager: Surya Narayanan Jayachandran
Cover Designer and Illustrator: Alice Premeau

Typeset by MPS Limited, Chennai, India

Dedication

I dedicate this volume to all those who savor the many important messages on the ways in which brain imaging has been oversold or otherwise misapplied, but who also believe that this general kind of message has itself been oversold: relish nuance.

Amir Raz

To my parents.

Robert T. Thibault

Contents

List of Contributors

Niels Birbaumer Institute of Medical Psychology and Behavioral Neurobiology, University of Tuebingen, Tuebingen, Germany; Wyss Center for Bio- and Neuroengineering, Geneva, Switzerland

Ricky Burns Max Planck Research Group for Neuroanatomy & Connectivity, Max Planck Institute for Human Cognitive and Brain Sciences, Leipzig, Germany

Henk R. Cremers Department of Clinical Psychology, University of Amsterdam, Amsterdam, The Netherlands

Lauren Dahl Cognitive Science, University of California Berkeley, Berkeley, CA, United States

Gustavo Deco Center for Brain and Cognition, Computational Neuroscience Group, Department of Information and Communication Technologies, Universitat Pompeu Fabra, Barcelona, Spain; Catalan Institution for Research and Advanced Studies (ICREA), Barcelona, Spain; Department of Neuropsychology, Max Planck Institute for Human Cognitive and Brain Sciences, Leipzig, Germany; School of Psychological Sciences, Monash University, Melbourne, Clayton, VIC, Australia

Gregory Donoghue Science of Learning Lecturer, Melbourne Graduate School of Education, University of Melbourne, Parkville, VIC, Australia

Jimmy Ghaziri Centre de Recherche du Centre Hospitalier de l'Université de Montréal, Montreal, QC, Canada; Département de Psychologie, Université du Québec à Montréal, Montreal, QC, Canada

Ian Gold Departments of Philosophy and Psychiatry, McGill University, Montreal, QC, Canada

Stevan Harnad Department of Psychology, Université du Québec à Montréal, Montreal, QC, Canada

David Haslacher Clinical Neurotechnology Laboratory, Neuroscience Research Center (NWFZ) & Department of Psychiatry and Psychotherapy, Charité – University Medicine Berlin, Germany; Applied Neurotechnology Laboratory, Department of Psychiatry and Psychotherapy, University Hospital of Tübingen, Tübingen, Germany

Philipp Haueis Berlin School of Mind and Brain, Humboldt Universitaet zu Berlin, Berlin, Germany; Institute of Philosophy, Bielefeld University, Bielefeld, Germany

Jared Cooney Horvath Graduate School of Education, University of Melbourne, Parkville, VIC, Australia

Alayar Kangarlu Department of Psychiatry, New York State Psychiatric Institute, Columbia University, New York, NY, United States

Laurence J. Kirmayer Division of Social & Transcultural Psychiatry, Department of Psychiatry, McGill University, Montreal, QC, Canada

Morten L. Kringelbach Department of Psychiatry, University of Oxford, Oxford, United Kingdom; Center for Music in the Brain, Department of Clinical Medicine, Aarhus University, Aarhus, Denmark

Michael Lifshitz Department of Anthropology, Stanford University, Palo Alto, CA, United States; Integrated Program in Neuroscience, McGill University, Montreal, QC, Canada

Scott O. Lilienfeld Department of Psychology, Emory University, Atlanta, Georgia, United States; University of Melbourne, Parkville, Australia

Erik Linstead Faculty of Computer Science, Schmid College of Science and Technology, Chapman University, Orange, CA, United States

Uri Maoz Assistant Professor of Computational Neuroscience Crean College of Health and Behavioral Sciences, Schmid College of Science and Technology, Institute for Interdisciplinary Brain and Behavioral Sciences, Chapman University, Orange, CA, United States; Visiting Assistant Professor of Department of Anesthesiology, David Geffen School of Medicine; Anderson School of Management; University of California Los Angeles, Los Angeles, CA, United States; Visiting Researcher in Neuroscience, California Institute of Technology, Pasadena, CA, United States

Daniel S. Margulies Max Planck Research Group for Neuroanatomy & Connectivity, Max Planck Institute for Human Cognitive and Brain Sciences, Leipzig, Germany

David Mehler School of Psychology, Cardiff University Brain Research Imaging Centre (CUBRIC), Cardiff, United Kingdom

Stephen J. Morse University of Pennsylvania Law School & Psychiatry Department, Philadelphia, PA, United States

Marcus R. Munafò UK Centre for Tobacco and Alcohol Studies, School of Psychological Science, University of Bristol, Bristol, United Kingdom; MRC Integrative Epidemiology Unit at the University of Bristol, Bristol, United Kingdom

Suresh Muthukumaraswamy School of Pharmacy, University of Auckland, Auckland, New Zealand

Jay A. Olson Department of Psychiatry, McGill University, Montreal, QC, Canada

Michael I. Posner University of Oregon, Eugene, OR, United States

Sheida Rabipour School of Psychology, University of Ottawa, Ottawa, ON, Canada

Aygul Rana Institute of Medical Psychology and Behavioral Neurobiology, University of Tübingen, Tübingen, Germany

Amir Raz Department(s) of Psychiatry, (Psychology, Neurology & Neurosurgery), McGill University and the Montreal Neurological Institute, Montreal, QC, Canada; Lady Davis Institute for Medical Research, Jewish General Hospital, Montreal, QC, Canada; Institute for Interdisciplinary Brain and Behavioral Sciences, Chapman University, Irvine, CA, United States

Sally Satel American Enterprise Institute, Washington, DC, United States

Amir Shmuel McConnell Brain Imaging Centre, Montreal Neurological Institute, Departments of Neurology, Neurosurgery, Physiology and Biomedical Engineering, McGill University, Montreal, QC, Canada

Surjo R. Soekadar Clinical Neurotechnology Laboratory, Neuroscience Research Center (NWFZ) & Department of Psychiatry and Psychotherapy, Charité — University Medicine Berlin, Germany; Applied Neurotechnology Laboratory, Department of Psychiatry and Psychotherapy, University Hospital of Tübingen, Tübingen, Germany

Robert T. Thibault Integrated Program in Neuroscience, McGill University, Montreal, QC, Canada

Evan Thompson Department of Philosophy, University of British Columbia, Vancouver, BC, Canada

Samuel Veissière Department of Psychiatry, Culture Mind and Brain Program, McGill University, Montreal, QC, Canada

Tor D. Wager Department of Psychology and Neuroscience and the Institute of Cognitive Science, University of Colorado, Denver, CO, United States

Tal Yarkoni Department of Psychology, University of Texas at Austin, Austin, TX, United States

Introductory Comments to Any Aspiring NeuroJedi: The Right Way to Read this Book

We wanted to have the term "NeuroJedi" in the title of our book, but some good people advised us that we may be hearing from George Lucas and his lawyers. By NeuroJedi, we wanted to allude to a good person who is trained to guard peace and justice in the neuroscience universe. As we wrote, collected, culled, and edited the chapters in this volume, we kept in mind and actively anticipated the human tendency for black-and-white thinking: either neuroimaging is good or it's bad. Accordingly, in putting together the materials contained in this book we wanted to help readers realize two important, albeit conflicting, tenets.

On the one hand, readers ought to realize that neuroscientists have obtained many wonderful insights by using brain imaging. On the other hand, this book highlights the overreach and tenuous nature of some of the claims emerging from reports describing neuroimaging findings. In academia, scholars often learn by pushing a position to an extreme, just to see how far it can go. Writing for a wide readership, however, calls for a different approach. Here we must be careful: we certainly don't want to give the impression that the whole imaging enterprise is bunk, because it isn't.

Imaging of the living human brain is a complicated and nuanced domain, rife with many a technical, statistical, and experimental tinge. As a graduate student, I was lucky to work with some of the researchers who had shaped the then-nascent field of cognitive neuroscience. One of the early influences on my career was the popular book *Images of Mind* by Michael I. Posner and Marcus E. Raichle. Later in my career, I had the pleasure of working closely with Mike Posner and the opportunity to interact with leading psychologists, physicists, computer scientists, mathematicians, statisticians, neurologists, psychiatrists, philosophers, linguists, anthropologists, sociologists, and other smart individuals with no title, who all weighed in on either the process or meaning of imaging the living human brain.

As a professor, I have either lectured on or listened to topics related to neuroimaging in some of the leading academic institutions. It took some time before it dawned on me that amongst experts, we often provide a quiet nod to, but rarely discuss, the painful shortcomings of brain imaging. Many reasons account for this trend, and perhaps this introduction isn't the best place to both enumerate and dwell on them. But the fact remains, newcomers to the field, experts from other domains and journalists who draw on imaging findings, or just curious folks who have not been sufficiently informed, frequently miss or blatantly ignore these lingering caveats.

Over the years, I have had the opportunity to intermingle with many students and uninitiated crowds, and engage in brief, leisurely, scheduled, and chance conversations on the topic of brain imaging with many a curious mind. The gist of these discussions almost always contained an element of indiscriminate reverence for brain scans by the nonexpert. Admittedly, I have been groomed to become a neuroimager. But after many cumulative years at the Weill Medical College of Cornell University, Columbia University Medical Center (College of Physicians and Surgeons), The New York Psychiatric Institute, The Brain Imaging Center at the Montreal Neurological Institute of McGill University—arguably some of the premier neuroimaging facilities on the East Coast—I have come to realize that we need to educate the masses by peppering some healthy cautions atop our intuitive fascination with brain imaging.

It gives me pleasure to have Robert T. Thibault, one of my senior doctoral students at McGill University, as a partner on this writing project. Robert started his way in my lab at McGill as a young undergraduate student. He has since grown to be a sophisticated critical thinker, including in the field of neuroimaging. From the harsh winters of Montreal to the sunny days of Southern California, Robert bore the main brunt of compiling this volume and seeing this project to fruition.

At the end of the day, critical thinking is what we advocate for in this book. Rather than seek to root out neuroimaging from our midst or portray it as bogus, we'd like for readers to develop an appreciation for this prickly technology—the rough with the smooth. Imaging of the living human brain forms a huge investment of time, resources, and effort by many intelligent scientists. We can learn a great deal from these research findings; however, we should grasp both the qualified merits and the relative drawbacks of neuroimaging as the field continues to evolve and the generation of Raz gives way to that of Thibault.

Amir Raz

Overview

Robert T. Thibault

This book is for anyone interested in brain science: for university students, for experts from fields that draw on brain imaging research, and for other curious minds. The chapters are short and nontechnical. They each introduce a key issue in the domain of human brain imaging and provide enough detail to appreciate the overarching concerns. By design, each chapter avoids detailed technicalities. For those interested in delving deeper into specific issues, at the end of each chapter you will find a list of recommended readings. While we recommend you read the book from beginning to end, each chapter can also be read as a standalone article. To lighten the book and keep things entertaining, we've included whimsical illustrations of a fellow aspiring NeuroJedi throughout.

This book surveys the field of human brain imaging through six sections. *Section I (Imaging brains: What for?)* outlines the wide-ranging fields that draw on neuroimaging—from cognitive science, psychiatry, and neurology to law and education. Experts from each of these fields highlight how much (or little) brain imaging has, and is expected to, contribute to their practice.

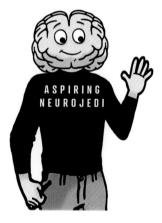

Section II (What are we measuring?) simplifies a topic often ceded to brain imaging specialists. This section explains how neuroimagers create colorful brain maps with functional magnetic resonance imaging (fMRI) and the nature of the brain waves recorded with electroencephalography (EEG). We discuss parameters that can influence brain imaging data—including posture, breathing, and muscle activity—and explain how to distinguish neural activity from random noise. *Section III (The devil's in the details)* approaches statistical issues with the nonstatistically minded at heart. It highlights how common analyses can inflate the positive tenor surrounding many brain imaging findings and outlines how we can overcome these concerns.

Section IV (Neuroimaging: Holy Grail or false prophet?) challenges our tendency to reduce complex phenomena to circumscribed brain processes and explores how this thinking colors our current state of knowledge. These chapters explore how we can overcome, and in some instances leverage, the popular belief that neuroscience alone can unveil the mechanisms behind human functioning. Such neuroreductionistic tendencies are not only common, but have also led many people to look for ways to train their brain. Subsequently, *Section V (Can we train the brain better?)* highlights the research surrounding the growing brain-training movement. Chapters in this section discuss brain stimulation, neurofeedback, computerized brain-training games, and mindfulness meditation.

Section VI (What next?) proposes ways to advance the field of brain imaging, from moving beyond single regions of interest and toward applying principles from network science as well as developing computational programs to model the dynamics of the entire brain. We then discuss advanced technologies that hold the potential to image at the cellular scale. This volume ends with a proposal for a multidisciplinary approach, which treats brain imaging as one method from a larger toolbox, to help understand and improve human behavior.

Whether you read these chapters on the subway, when taking a break from work, or before turning off the lights at night, we hope the material comes through as engaging and insightful. Above all, we hope that this book impacts not only *what* you think about human brain imaging, but rather, *how* you think about it.

Neuroskepticism: questioning the brain as symbol and selling-point

Neuroskeptic, Pseudonymous blogger, Discover Magazine

It was nearly 10 years ago that I put on the mask of pseudonymity and began writing a blog called "Neuroskeptic." At that time I was a mere PhD student and my blog, in the first couple of years, was hardly read. So I was pleased and honored to find myself, a decade later, being invited to write an introduction to a book on "The Dark Side of Brain Imaging." It has been wonderful to see the growth over time of what I would call a critical or skeptical approach to neuroscience, something I found was lacking 10 years ago (hence why I took up the challenge). I do not think that a book like this would have been possible back then. This is not, of course, to suggest that I was the first neuroskeptic,[1] but a decade ago, there did not seem to be the level of awareness of the need to keep a level head when it comes to the brain that we now have today.

So what has happened over the past 10 years to generate this growth in skepticism? Has brain science somehow degenerated, and become more deserving of criticism? On the contrary, in my view, many of the problems that troubled me about my field, as a neuroscience PhD student, have largely been solved. Neuroscience has benefited from methodological refinement and increased emphasis on statistical rigor. I would say that the neuroscience papers published today are generally far stronger than when I started blogging.

There have, certainly, been a number of well-publicized "scandals" in neuroscience, especially surrounding functional MRI (fMRI), which is the leading method for measuring neural activity. We've had the "voodoo" scandal [1], the "dead salmon" affair [2] and, more recently, the "cluster failure" controversy [3]. But cognitive neuroscience and fMRI research has emerged stronger after each one. Each of these scandals centered around a particular statistical pitfall or flaw which was discovered to have affected lots of fMRI studies. But the flaws, once identified, proved easy to fix. And while it is true that there are still, depressingly, papers published today that fall prey to these same errors, the field as a whole has moved pass them.

[1] For example, one of my main inspirations was another pseudonymous blogger, The Neurocritic (http://neurocritic.blogspot.com).

Neuroscience is also getting bigger—in terms of sample sizes (chapter 12). Thanks to data sharing initiatives such as the Human Connectome Project, neuroscientists are now routinely carrying out brain scanning studies with several hundreds, or even more than a thousand, brains. This just didn't happen in the past. Larger samples bring some challenges of their own, but they translate directly to more robust results. Lastly, there is a growing awareness of something I wrote about in my very first post—the distorting effect of scientists' desire to find "positive" results. The "replication crisis" (chapter 11), which began about 5 years ago in psychology, is also making itself felt in the field of neuroscience.

So if neuroscience isn't getting worse, why is neuroskepticism growing? I think the answer to this is simple: The brain has taken over the wider culture.

Already 10 years ago, neuroscience was routinely over-hyped in the media, but if things were bad then, the past decade has seen neuro-nonsense grow into a thriving industry (chapter 22).

In 2007, someone coined the term "Neuroleadership"—as in, how to be a brain-based boss. Just a silly neologism? Maybe, but in 2018, the NeuroLeadership Institute has 70 employees and an annual revenue of $12 million. If leadership's not for you, don't worry: you can spend thousands of dollars in courses on brain-based parenting, brain-based teaching (chapter 6), brain-based life coaching and even brain-based storytelling. This is not to mention the global success of brain training games (chapter 20). Neuroscience has also become central to our conversations. Consider the worry over whether Facebook or smartphones are causing too much dopamine release, or the increasing use of neuroscience in the courtroom (chapter 5).

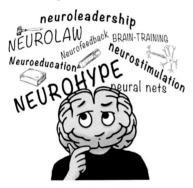

I think it is this expansion of popular (or, less kindly, vulgar) neuroscience that has brought with it an expansion of neuroskepticism—and a good thing too. Because, speaking as a neuroscientist, I do not think that we know nearly enough about the brain to be able to give advice on parenting, leadership, or social issues. Not yet. Perhaps the day will come that a neuroscientist is able to know more about a child than their own parent, or more about a company than its own CEO; but that day has not yet come.

I am not saying that neuroscience will never be able to speak to everyday issues. I believe that the brain is the basis for all our thoughts and behaviors. In principle, therefore, if we knew enough about the brain, we would be able to predict and control behavior—but the devil is in the details. We don't currently know the details well enough to be able to say anything useful about the behavior of most people.

Most neuroscientists are well aware of the limitations of their field which is why—with a few unfortunate exceptions—it is not neuroscientists who are responsible for neuro-hype. Where, then, does it come from? I'm really not sure. Perhaps this is just the age of the brain. In 30 years, as neuroscience has matured, popular culture will probably have moved on to worship something else.

Section I

Imaging brains: What for?

Can neuroimaging reveal how the brain thinks?

1

Stevan Harnad

There is no doubt about the usefulness of neuroimaging (pictures of brain structure and brain activity) in clinical neurology (e.g., brain injuries, brain dysfunction). The question here is whether neuroimaging can help us understand and explain how the normal brain works [1]. That is the territory of cognitive science, a new field (or family of fields, including psychology, neuroscience, ethology, computer science, linguistics, and philosophy) whose goal is to explain "cognition." Cognition means whatever is going on in our heads while doing whatever we are doing. It's almost synonymous with "thinking" [2].

Descartes is famous for his "cogito ergo sum": "I think therefore I am." The "therefore I am" part is for philosophers to worry about, but the "I think" part is about what is going on in our brains. We all know what it feels like to think. Descartes pointed out that you can doubt just about everything—what people tell us (maybe they're lying), whether other people think (maybe they're just zombies), what science tells us (maybe tomorrow apples will fall up instead of down), what our eyes tell us (maybe I'm hallucinating it all)—but you can't doubt that you're thinking, when you're thinking.

Cognitive science is about what is really happening in your brain when you're thinking. What is thinking? You can't answer that with the cogito. The cogito just tells you that it happens when it happens. Cognitive science is trying to find out what is actually happening when it happens. You would think that when you're thinking, you know what's happening, and so you can tell us. That's called "intro-spection." But it doesn't work. Introspection can tell you *when* you're thinking, what you're thinking *about*, and what it *feels like* to be thinking. But it can't tell what thinking is. It can't tell you how your brain is actually doing it.

We have other organs besides the brain: the heart, stomach, liver, kidneys, and lungs. Let's call their functions "vegetative," in contrast to cognitive functions. Bioimaging of vegetative function is also useful for clinical purposes. But heart imaging is useful not only in diagnosing but also even in repairing heart malfunc-tion: If it were not for the fact that we already know most of *how* the heart does what it does (pump blood) from centuries of basic research on the anatomy, physio-logy, and biochemistry of the heart, the newly invented capability of visualizing the heart would have been able to fast-forward us there today. The reason is simple. We can visualize what hearts do because vegetative functions, such as pumping blood—or even regulating heart rate or blood pressure, which are done by the brain

Casting Light on the Dark Side of Brain Imaging. DOI: https://doi.org/10.1016/B978-0-12-816179-1.00001-3

rather than the heart—can be observed directly. The brain has vegetative functions too, and neuroimaging will no doubt be helpful in understanding those better too. But what about understanding cognitive functions?

The heart pumps blood. What does the brain "pump" when it is performing cognitive rather than vegetative functions? Alan Turing (who was certainly not a brain scientist) pointed out the simple answer: "Cognizing" is whatever our brain is doing when we (the organisms who have the brain) are doing the kinds of things we call cognitive rather than vegetative [3]. Our brains are cognizing when they are perceiving, recognizing, remembering, reasoning, learning, speaking, or understanding—but not when they are raising or lowering our blood pressure or temperature, dilating our pupils, maintaining our balance, making us feel hungry or keeping us breathing. In fact, everything we do voluntarily rather than automatically or reflexively is cognizing.

In other words, what our brain pumps (cognitively speaking) is whatever we do voluntarily, but not only what we actually do, but also what we are *able* to do: The brain generates our cognitive capacity—which Turing, in his day, called our *intelligence*. Turing also had a hypothesis about *how* the brain generates our intelligence: through computation. Turing was one of the coinventors of the computer as well as one of the fathers of what is now called "artificial intelligence" but might as well have been called *artificial cognition*. He demonstrated that computation—which is the manipulation of symbols (e.g., 0 and 1) based on formal rules called "algorithms"—is virtually omnipotent: a computer can do just about anything that any "machine" in the universe, actual or possible, physical or biological, can do.

This is not the end of the story, but it brings us immediately to an explanation of why neuroimaging cannot reveal how the brain is generating cognitive function: It is for the very same reason that cyber-imaging cannot reveal what software a computer is running. We can observe what the computer is doing on the outside—its inputs and outputs—but that does not tell us what program (algorithm) it is executing. To figure out what algorithm a computer is executing to generate its outputs in response to its inputs, it does not help to observe what is going on inside the computer either. Discovering the algorithm requires another kind of creativity, a little more like what was going on in Newton's brain to determine what makes apples fall to earth. Newton did not figure that out by observing apple or earth imaging of what happens inside the apple or inside the earth when an apple falls.

Before cognitive science, experimental psychologists had hoped to be able to figure out how the brain does what it does by first studying what it can do, in other words studying its behavior, its outputs in response to its inputs. They hoped to combine these behavioral data with anatomical, physiological, and biochemical data on what goes on inside the brain, mostly through experiments on nonhuman animals (many of them at the cost of great pain and suffering to the animals). But while they studied these neurobiological correlates of animal behavior, psychologists and philosophers kept dreaming of a "cerebroscope" that would allow them to study the neurobiological correlates of human behavior in live, behaving human beings [4]. The advent of neuroimaging seemed to realize their dreams. But several subsequent decades have shown that the goal—to discover and explain how the brain does what it does (which is all the things that humans can do) remains as distant as before.

We fill journal upon journal with articles on the brain correlates of behavior and cognition: where and when in the brain the activity occurs when we are cognizing. But "where" and "when" stubbornly keeps refusing to reveal *how* those brain correlates generate our cognition and the behavior. The reports of the correlations are as fascinating and as addictive as horoscopes—but they are about equally explanatory.

Is the lack of progress because we have not been imaging and correlating long enough? Is it because Turing was right, that we are looking for the algorithms, and you can't find those by observing what's going on inside? Or is it because cognitive science still lacks its Newton to make sense of it all?

I don't know the answer, but let me close by considering yet another layer of complexity: Although Turing is surely right about the universal power of computation, it does not follow that all there is in the world is computation. Electricity is not computation. Chemistry is not computation. Heat is not computation. Movement is not computation. Pumping blood is not computation. They can all be simulated, computationally, by computation. But the simulations do not have the electrical, chemical, and other dynamic properties of the real thing. Why should it be different with cognition? What we are looking for, when we are trying to figure out how the brain cognizes, is a causal mechanism. The causal mechanism may well be dynamic, like apples falling, rather than computational (though like falling apples, it can be simulated computationally). Yet the causal mechanism can't be just vegetative either. Cognizing is not just moving.

So my bet is that what cognitive science needs much more than cerebroscopes is its share of Newtons

Additional readings

Aue T, Lavelle LA, Cacioppo JT. Great expectations: what can fMRI research tell us about psychological phenomena? Int J Psychophysiol 2009;73(1):10−16.

Coltheart M. Perhaps functional neuroimaging has not told us anything about the mind (so far). Cortex 2006;42(3):422−7.

de Zubicaray G. Strong inference in functional neuroimaging. Aust J Psychol 2012;64 (1):19−28.

Farah MJ. Brain images, babies, and bathwater: critiquing critiques of functional neuroimaging. Hast Center Rep 2014;44(s2).

Levin Y, Aharon I. What's on your mind? A brain scan won't tell. Rev Philos Psychol 2011;2(4):699−722.

Ozdemir M. Controversial science of brain imaging. Sci Am Blog 2012; (2012).

Page MP. What can't functional neuroimaging tell the cognitive psychologist? Cortex 2006;42(3):428−43.

Wright J. The analysis of data and the evidential scope of neuroimaging results. Br J Philos Sci 2017.

Is addiction a brain disease?

2

Scott O. Lilienfeld and Sally Satel

> *If we take in our hand any volume; of divinity or school metaphysics, for instance;*
> *let us ask, Does it contain any abstract reasoning concerning quantity or number?*
> *"No. Does it contain any experimental reasoning concerning matter of fact and*
> *existence?" No. Commit it then to the flames: for it can contain nothing but*
> *sophistry and illusion (Hume, 1748, p. 165) [1].*

After reading a draft of a paper, physicist Wolfgang Pauli purportedly exclaimed, "Es ist nicht einmal falsch!" ("It is not even wrong!") [2]. Pauli's quip reminds us that some scientific assertions are so nebulous that they do not have the virtue of being refutable, even in principle. Following the lead of Sir Karl Popper [3], many philosophers of science would concur that claims that could never be falsified given any conceivable set of data are unscientific. Philosopher David Hume made a similar point in our opening quotation: A proposition that does not generate measurable predictions is scientifically meaningless: It should be committed to the flames.

In this commentary, we advance a heretical position: The proposition that addictions are brain diseases is fundamentally unscientific. In the words of Pauli, it is not even wrong. To be more precise, some aspects of the brain disease claim are unfalsifiable whereas others are falsifiable; and those aspects that are falsifiable have now been falsified.

The familiar meme that addictions are brain diseases took hold in the mid-1990s, coinciding with the advent of modern brain imaging techniques, especially positron emission tomography (PET) and functional magnetic resonance imaging (fMRI). In 1997 Alan Leshner, then head of the National Institute on Drug Abuse (NIDA), authored an influential article in the prestigious journal *Science* entitled "Addiction is a Brain Disease, and It Matters" [4]. Leshner staked out a bold position on addiction, describing it as "a chronic, relapsing brain disorder characterized by compulsive drug seeking" (p. 45). He argued that chronic use of psychoactive substances often damages brain circuitry to the extent that the capacity to resist drug use is severely impaired. Likening addiction to Alzheimer's disease, Leshner contended that the addicted require medical treatment. Many prominent figures and public officials, including Nora Volkow, current head of NIDA, and former

Casting Light on the Dark Side of Brain Imaging. DOI: https://doi.org/10.1016/B978-0-12-816179-1.00014-1

Surgeon General Vivek Murthy, have since embraced and promoted the brain disease framework of addiction [5−7] as have scores of addiction treatment centers. Many brain imaging investigators now unabashedly invoke this model as a justification for their research.

Several key tenets of the brain disease model of addiction are vague, rendering them challenging, if not impossible, to test. Nevertheless, this model appears to comprise three key assertions: (1) addictions are traceable to dysfunctions in brain circuitry; (2) addictions are chronic and relapsing conditions; and (3) addicts' brains are sufficiently compromised that they have largely lost the capacity to refrain from pathological use. Let's examine each of these propositions in turn.

The NIDA website asserts that addiction is "a brain disease because drugs change the brain; they change its structure and how it works" [8]. The finding that chronic substance use changes the brain has been supported by brain imaging studies. Data show that the brains of addicted individuals tend to display diminished activity in regions linked to inhibitory control, such as the orbitofrontal cortex and cingulate gyrus [9]. Nevertheless, such findings are in no way specific to addiction. For example, brain imaging studies demonstrate that reading alters brain activity, and that extended juggling alters brain structure [10,11]. In fact, the finding that prolonged substance use alters brain activity as revealed by PET and fMRI scanning is entirely unsurprising, even trivial, from a neuroscientific standpoint. Given that all behaviors are mediated by brain functioning, the finding that chronic substance use affects the brain is barely more than a self-evident scientific truism [12].

Indeed, it is hard to envision precisely what kind of neuroscientific findings could even be invoked to falsify the assertion that addictions are rooted in brain functioning. For example, plentiful data demonstrate that psychosocial variables, such as life stressors, peer influences, neighborhood factors, and availability of substances, play key roles in addiction risk, suggesting that a primary or even exclusive focus on a disordered brain as the principal culprit in addiction is misplaced [13]. In response, some brain disease enthusiasts have argued that the roles of social and psychological factors are actually consistent with the brain disease model, because these variables ultimately exert their influence via the brain.

This rhetorical ploy essentially renders the brain disease model unfalsifiable, because all psychological factors, including basic learning processes, necessarily affect the brain at some level [14]. Moreover, this tactic sidesteps the point that the brain is merely one lens of analysis among many for explaining addiction, and not necessarily the most important for intervention or prevention. Finally, extending this analysis to its (il)logical conclusion, one could just as legitimately contend that these findings are consistent with an "atomic model" of addiction given that all psychosocial variables influence the brain's atoms. (But why stop there? We could also entertain a quark model of addiction, for instance).

Seeking to account for complex phenomena in terms of their lower-order constituents—an approach that philosophers term *explanatory reductionism* (see Chapter 14)—is not always a helpful scientific strategy [15]. Imagine that jumbo jets kept blowing up in midair during the summer because the airlines routinely left them sitting on tarmacs in scorching heat for hours prior to take-off. An analysis of each plane's 3 million-plus parts in an effort to detect the cause of the explosions would be fruitless, because the plane's design and construction are not at fault. It would be equally misleading to conceptualize the cause of the explosions as "an airplane parts problem" on the grounds that the excessive heat interacts with the plane's subcomponents.

Unquestionably, addictions are brain diseases from the perspective of *one* lens of analysis, namely, neuroimaging and neuroscience more generally. But addictions are every bit as much motivational diseases, personality diseases, social diseases, cultural diseases, and so on. There is, thus, scant scientific or logical justification for privileging one lens of analysis, such as the lens of neuroimaging, above all others [16]. A full understanding of the causes, treatment, and prevention of addiction will require improved knowledge of its brain-based causes, and neuroimaging will almost surely assist us in this endeavor. But it will also require better knowledge of other contributors, including learning history, motivation, personality traits, and the social and cultural setting of addiction. Notably, in his 1997 article, Leshner acknowledged that "Addiction is not just a brain disease... It is a brain disease for which the social contexts in which it has both developed and is expressed are critically important" (p. 46). Regrettably, this caveat appears to have been largely ignored by scholars.

What, now, about the assertion that addictions are chronic, relapsing conditions? Here, the data are unequivocal. In controlled studies, many or most addicts manage to quit on their own, without formal treatment [17,18]. In our experience, many addiction practitioners and researchers are skeptical of these data. We suspect they have fallen prey to the *clinician's illusion*, the tendency to overestimate the persistence of psychological conditions over time. After all, practitioners routinely encounter patients who fail to improve and rarely encounter patients who improve on their own. This is no surprise, as people who recover rarely need treatment or volunteer as addiction research participants [19].

A final cornerstone of the brain disease model is that addicts' brains are so badly damaged that their owners have lost the capacity to refrain from use. Here the model possesses a kernel of truth insofar as brain imaging studies indicate that prolonged substance use sometimes damages brain regions mediating impulse control. As a consequence, addicts often find it difficult to refrain from use. Still, there is clear evidence that most or all people with long-standing substance addictions retain the capacity to curtail use in the presence of external incentives.

For example, during the Vietnam War, between 10% and 25% of American GI's were addicted to high-grade heroin. Yet, once they returned home, heroin apparently lost its appeal, and most recovered. Heroin helped soldiers endure war-time's alternating bouts of boredom and terror, but stateside, where use was a crime and civilian life took precedence, its allure faded [20].

Let's further consider the commonly invoked comparison of addictions with neurological diseases, such as Alzheimer's disease. If one held a gun to the head of a person addicted to alcohol and threatened to shoot her if she consumed another drink, she could comply with this demand—and the odds are high that she would. In contrast, pointing a gun to the head of a patient with Alzheimer's disease and threatening to shoot her unless her memory improved would be futile. The analogy between addictions and classic neurological illnesses fails [12].

Further undercutting the notion that brain changes invariably lead to drug consumption is the extent to which users' expectation of the drug's pending effect influence their behavior. Research using *balanced placebo designs* suggests that among individuals with alcohol use disorder (formerly called alcoholism), the decision to drink is driven largely by beliefs about what they are consuming. In these designs, participants are randomly assigned to one of four conditions, in which they ingest (1) an alcoholic drink and are informed correctly that it contains alcohol, (2) a placebo drink (one that does not contain alcohol but is mixed to taste like alcohol) and are informed correctly that it does not contain alcohol, (3) an alcoholic drink but are informed incorrectly that it does not contain alcohol, or (4) a placebo drink but are informed incorrectly that it contains alcohol.

Data reveal that alcoholics assigned to condition (3) often refrain from drinking, but that those assigned to condition (4) frequently fail to do so [21]. At least with respect to alcohol, these results raise serious questions concerning the assumption that addicts' altered brain physiology renders them incapable of stopping use. The results also underscore the importance of examining lenses of analyses in addition to the brain, in this case a psychological perspective that incorporates addicts' expectations [22].

Lastly, people consume drugs and alcohol for psychological reasons. Addicted individuals variously describe the value of substances in quelling anxiety, feelings of emptiness, self-loathing, and boredom. They can give meaningful responses to the question: Why do you use drugs? An Alzheimer's patient, in contrast, would find the questions (assuming that she could understand them)—Why is your cognition failing? Why do you allow it to fail?—to be incoherent. To be sure, a neurobiologist could explain the processes associated with her brain degeneration, but she would never think to explain her condition in psychological terms.

So, even if the brain disease model is logically and scientifically indefensible, is it useful? In at least three ways, the answer appears to be no. First, this model has not pointed scientists toward beneficial interventions. The few modestly effective treatments for addiction, such as naloxone (which blocks the action of the brain's endogenous opioids), were developed long before the full-scale advent of modern brain imaging methods and the conceptualization of addiction as a brain affliction [23]. In addition, the brain disease model prioritizes medication over psychosocial interventions, which are essential to recovery. *Contingency management*, in which addicts receive tangible rewards for staying off drugs, has been found to be effective in many controlled studies [24,25]. Second, although advocates of the brain disease model often maintain that it reduces stigma, the evidence is mixed. Studies suggest that although informing alcoholics that their substance use is attributable to a brain disease may alleviate self-blame, it diminishes their belief that they can control their drinking [26]. Third the brain disease model does little to explain dramatic shifts in the societal prevalence of addictions. As we write this essay, the United States is in the midst of the most lethal opioid epidemic in its history. Yet, Americans' brains have not changed. Instead, what has changed is an increased

availability of diverted pain medica-
tions, combined with the despair and
economic dislocation created by dein-
dustrialization and a growing sense
among many that the American Dream
is no longer attainable [27,28].

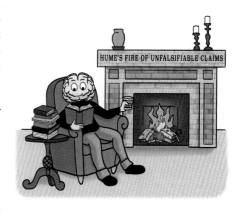

In sum, the brain disease model of
addiction is little more than a vague met-
aphor, despite concerted efforts to confirm it with neuroimaging. It is unhelpful
at best and misleading at worst. The
model hinges on a presupposition—that
addictions are diseases of the brain—that
is unfalsifiable and essentially devoid of scientific content. In this regard, it is not even
wrong. Further, addicts' capacity for choice-making, albeit at times compromised, is
by no means obliterated in the face of demonstrable brain changes. It is high time that
we commit this model to the flames.

Additional readings

A brief and accessible review of the brain disease model of addiction, with a particular focus
   on the data on the effects of methamphetamine on the brain: Grifell M, Hart CL. Is drug
   addiction a brain disease? This popular claim lacks evidence and leads to poor policy.
   Am Sci 2018;106:160−7.
Good survey of the evidence for brain disease model, including its questionable track record
   for generating novel and effective interventions: Hall W, Carter A, Forlini C. The brain
   disease model of addiction: is it supported by the evidence and has it delivered on its
   promises? Lancet Psychiatr 2015;2:105−10.

How brain imaging takes psychiatry for a ride

Surjo R. Soekadar and David Haslacher

One out of every four people seeks psychiatric or psychological support. They do so because they experience patterns of behavior and thought that cause them significant distress or functional impairment. Researchers estimated that mental disorders account for 32.4% of years lived with disability and 13.0% of disability-adjusted life-years worldwide [1]. This prevalence translates to a global economic burden of approximately 8.5 trillion USD each year. During my daily routine as a psychiatrist the meaning of this unimaginable number becomes tangible in the anxiety and despair of people who, in some cases, have lost everything, from their jobs to their relationships and sometimes even their will to live. Faced with the unvarnished reality and hardship of mental disorders, almost every clinician would immediately endorse a technical tool that quickly identifies the cause of a person's emotional turmoil, psychotic rage, inner emptiness, or serious forgetfulness. Many of us assume that once we know the cause, we'll know how to fix it.

Consequently the development of brain imaging tools to directly or indirectly image the structure and function of the nervous system has catalyzed hopes that science would finally identify the substrate of mental disorders, such as major depression or schizophrenia [2]. Once identified, we could be able to understand and specifically target them. And indeed, over the years, the applied methods became more and more sophisticated offering an ever increasing resolution and imaging performance.

However, none of these methods can yet identify the individual substrate of a mental disorder. It is still impossible to predict and characterize a mental disorder solely based on brain imaging. Up until now, brain imaging has yielded very limited impact on psychiatric treatments, and there is currently no evidence that we could use brain imaging to diagnose a mental disorder in the near future (even if some physicians, who typically make a fortune with brain imaging, claim they can do so).

In my clinical routine, brain imaging is mainly used to rule out "organic" causes for mental health problems, such as head trauma, stroke, tumors, seizure disorders, or previous toxin exposure. But why aren't we using brain scans to diagnose depression, posttraumatic stress disorder (PTSD), obsessive–compulsive disorder (OCD), or schizophrenia? Isn't depression just an under-activation of the left

Casting Light on the Dark Side of Brain Imaging. DOI: https://doi.org/10.1016/B978-0-12-816179-1.00002-5

dorsolateral prefrontal cortex, as countless lifestyle magazines report? Isn't an addiction merely a dysregulation of the nucleus accumbens, a key area of the reward system? The answer is *probably not*.

There are good reasons to doubt that brain imaging will play any major role in psychiatric diagnosis in the near future. The main reasons relate to the following three fundamental issues that are partly rooted in the history of psychiatric diagnostics and the nature of brain imaging.

1. *The specific substrate and mechanisms of behavioral or mental patterns underlying mental disorders are largely unknown. Such knowledge would be important to define distinct disease categories that are based on traceable and verifiable mechanisms.*

The first nosological scheme for psychiatric disorders was proposed by Emil Kraepelin (1856–1926), who postulated that each nosological entity (disease or illness) is signified by the concurrence of *etiology* (set of causes), *neuropathology* (characteristic alterations of the nervous system), and *clinical course*. However, due to lack of biological measures providing a consistent pathophysiological model for the proposed psychiatric entities, clinicians currently base diagnosis of most mental disorders on *clinical symptom observation* and the *course of disease*.

For example, to be diagnosed with depression, a patient must express at least two of three main symptoms and three of seven cosymptoms. This diagnostic system can lead to the awkward situation that two people sharing almost no clinical symptoms receive the same diagnosis. Moreover, some clinical symptoms can occur across different disorders, such as emotional instability, anxiety, impulsivity, or delusions, which can lead to the opposite problem—depending on the course of disease or cooccurrence with other symptoms, the same symptom can result in a different diagnosis.

While the first editions of the American Psychiatric Association's (APA's) Diagnostic and Statistical Manual of Mental Disorders (DSM) still adhered to explicit disease models as proposed by Kraepelin, the DSM-III (1980) abandoned this ambition and replaced the term *disease* by the term *disorder*. Since the first edition of the DSM that was released in 1952, the number of diagnoses multiplied from 106 to almost 300 in the DSM-5.

Numerous scientific studies identify the brain correlates of various behavioral and mental patterns and seem to justify this ever-expanding taxonomy. But is it so surprising that distinct behaviors or mental patterns have a distinct correlate in the structure or function of the nervous system?

Certainly, identifying such correlates is important, but framing such findings as neuropathological substrates and proof of a mental disorder is misleading and dangerous. It will promote further inflation of diagnoses that may create millions of newly mislabeled "patients," resulting in unnecessary and potentially harmful treatments, stigma, and wasteful misallocation of scarce resources [3].

Given their obvious limitations, it is very likely that the diagnostic manuals will be stepwise modified and finally replaced by a neuroscience-based nosological system in which each category relates to a specific pathomechanism as originally intended by Emil Kraepelin.

The Research Domain Criteria (RDoC) framework introduced by the National Institute of Mental Health (NIMH), which incorporates multiple dimensions, such as behavior, thought patterns, neurobiological measures, and genetics, may become a basis or blueprint for such a system. In contrast to current models of mental disorders, the RDoC approach incorporates measures of magnitude and severity centered around five broad domains of psychological function (cognitive systems, positive valence systems, negative valence systems, arousal-regulatory systems, and social processes).

Over the decades the DSM classification system has become deeply integrated into the healthcare system in terms of insurance, clinical organization, and disease management. Thus we can imagine that the DSM-style systems and neuroscience-based frameworks will run in parallel for some time. A general obstacle for the broad implementation of neuroscience-based frameworks for mental disorders, however, is its dependence on technologies (e.g., for tracking behavioral patterns, assessing neurobiological measures) that are currently only available in the more economically developed countries.

2. *Brain imaging can only depict correlative and not causal relationships between the brain and behavioral or mental patterns that cause distress or impairment of personal functioning.*

Since the early 20th century, brain imaging along with the discovery of antipsychotic and antidepressant drugs supported the assumption that mental disorders have a distinct biological substrate. For instance, in 1955, Gerd Huber discovered an enlargement of the third ventricle (a brain cavity filled with cerebrospinal fluid) in people who were newly diagnosed with schizophrenia [4]—a finding that some researchers and clinicians used as a strong argument against nonbiomedical (social) models of schizophrenia. There is no doubt that, since the 1950s, brain imaging provided invaluable insights for a better understanding of how behavioral and mental patterns relate to brain structure and function. However, these relationships are of *purely correlative nature*. Moreover, many such reported relationships are biased by statistical errors (see Section III: The Devil's in the Details).

Despite these critical limitations of brain imaging, the idea persists that brain imaging reflects the *neural substrate* of a specific mental disorder (see point 1) or brain function. Until researchers show that purposefully modifying a specific *neural substrate* alters a given behavior or mental state, our expectations and hopes that brain imaging will contribute to psychiatric diagnostics and better psychiatric treatments will remain unfulfilled.

A possible way to overcome this second fundamental problem is to combine brain imaging with a means to directly modify brain activity; for example, using invasive or noninvasive brain stimulation. Combining such approaches would allow researchers to demonstrate a *causal link* between neural activity, brain function and behavior [5,6]. Though technically very challenging, recent advances allowing for real-time functional imaging pave the way to advance such setups toward closed-loop stimulation and neurofeedback paradigms. Besides further elucidating brain—behavior relationships, these approaches may also prove useful in promoting functional and structural neuroplasticity, which in turn, could foster neural recovery and mental health [7].

3. *The way most brain imaging results originate (by contrasting activation patterns across patients and healthy controls performing various behavioral or cognitive tasks) inherently limits their specificity and sensitivity in detecting a mental disorder.*

Brain activity is extremely variable from person to person, even for similar cognitive processes. Given that psychiatrists distinguish some mental disorders based on their clinical course, acquiring brain images at a single time point is likely insufficient to capture the brain disorder investigated. This problem amplifies when we take into account that many of the proposed disease categories (e.g., schizophrenia or depression) may only represent the common final pathway of very different brain disorders. Another problem is that many patients (approximately 15%−20%) suffer from more than one disorder, making it challenging to separate these disorders by looking at brain imaging results.

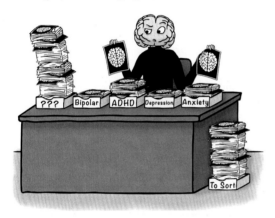

Moreover, brain imaging protocols and devices vary across acquisition sites, which in turn, creates a problem of *standardization*. Meta-analyses of brain imaging studies show that mental disorders, which the DSM-5 differentiates, actually share the same areas of activation. Think about brain areas such as the amygdala or insula, which are shown to be over-activated across various disorders such as generalized anxiety disorder, PTSD, OCD, and social phobia. Despite plenty of evidence that the imaging techniques employed are reliable, such studies add little to what is already known. On the contrary, they create the impression of novelty, when in fact no consistent discrimination pattern for a specific brain function or brain disorder was provided.

Researchers could improve the sensitivity and specificity of brain imaging−based diagnostics by employing mathematical and statistical models which can be causally tested via noninvasive brain stimulation. As a second step, they could use these models to purposefully shift brain states toward desirable directions using advanced brain activity−informed stimulation protocols.

Looking to the future, we may be able to resolve the three abovementioned core issues. New computational tools and multivariate statistical approaches show some promise for identifying specific mental disorders [8]. However, it seems that we need a fundamentally different approach to advance brain imaging to the point of serving as a useful tool in mental health diagnostics. Admittedly the task is incredibly challenging, if not impossible, as the mental disorders currently listed in the DSM-5 may be in contradiction with categorizations derived from brain imaging or other neurobiological measures.

Certainly, ignoring the fundamental problems raised earlier may be very convenient or even profitable for some neuroscientists and clinical psychiatrists. But given the hundreds of millions of dollars that have been spent on brain imaging over many decades and the very limited impact they have had on clinical psychiatry, it is our responsibility to effectively tackle these issues now. Only then will both brain imaging and psychiatry reach their full potential for improving mental health and helping those who seek psychiatric or psychological support.

Additional readings

Farah MJ, Gillihan SJ. The puzzle of neuroimaging and psychiatric diagnosis: technology and nosology in an evolving discipline. AJOB Neurosci 2012;3:31—41.

Hyman SE. The diagnosis of mental disorders: the problem of reification. Annu Rev Clin Psychol 2010;6:155—79.

Linden DE. The challenges and promise of neuroimaging in psychiatry. Neuron 2012;73 (1):8—22.

Brain–computer interfaces for communication in paralysis

4

Niels Birbaumer and Aygul Rana

Several neurodegenerative diseases can attack the peripheral and central motor system—amyotrophic lateral sclerosis (ALS), Parkinson's disease, multiple sclerosis, and Guillain−Barré syndrome, to name just a few. In later stages of these diseases, patients lose their ability to communicate and interact with the world in traditional ways. While their brain functions remain intact, they lose voluntary control over their body. To improve the quality of life of these patients, brain−computer interfaces (BCIs) appear to be the most promising technologies. BCIs translate brain activity into a command for an external device in order to perform a particular function; for example, to control a prosthetic or to speak. A prime example of a BCI includes an electroencephalogram (EEG) that records the alpha rhythm (13−15 Hz) over the motor cortex in stroke patients and gives a command to an artificial support that can help mobilize a paralyzed arm. Other BCIs are used to train participants to amplify or reduce certain brain activities in a process called neurofeedback. Other BCIs can use machine learning algorithms to passively distinguish between two or more brain states. This chapter focuses on using BCIs to allow completely paralyzed patients to communicate.

Brain−computer interfaces in paralysis

Our research group works primarily with patients suffering from the neurodegenerative disease called ALS, or Lou Gehrig's disease. ALS is a progressive motor disease without a known cause. It dramatically reduces the motor function of those afflicted but has no major impact on sensory and cognitive functions [1]. The disease initially affects respiration and as it progresses, patients lose control of their muscles. Currently, there is no treatment available for ALS. Thus at the later stage of the disease, patients need to make a difficult decision between artificial respiration and tube feeding or death due to suffocation.

In a clinical setting, patients are classified into one of two states, namely locked-in state (LIS), where patients maintain residual control over some muscles, and completely LIS (CLIS), where muscular control is completely absent. ALS patients

Casting Light on the Dark Side of Brain Imaging. DOI: https://doi.org/10.1016/B978-0-12-816179-1.00003-7

in CLIS are unable to communicate in normal ways as they lack voluntary control over their muscles. Although they have no control over their body, similar to some patients in a minimally conscious state, evidence suggests that their brain continues to function [2].

The first successful BCI on two severely, but not completely, paralyzed ALS patients by Birbaumer et al. [3] used a type of brain wave known as slow cortical potentials (negative or positive polarizations of the EEG that last up to several seconds). The patients learned to manipulate these brain waves voluntarily and used them for selecting letters presented on a computer screen. Patients were first trained over a period of several weeks to control their slow cortical potentials with a neurofeedback procedure. Later, having mastered self-control of their brain waves, they selected letters and formed words on a computer screen with a simple letter speller.

Patients who have remaining control of their eyes can communicate with devices that track their eye movements and select letters or commands on a computer screen. While the patients in Birbaumer et al. [3] had some remaining muscular control and eye control, one of them, during BCI use over several years, required the BCI during the periods of exhaustion but was, from time to time, still able to clearly answer "yes" and "no" with facial muscles. Some patients, who become tired from eye control (most of whom showed only minimal voluntary control over gaze) and make many errors, prefer a BCI [4,5].

In 2007, Birbaumer and his group submitted a meta-analysis of BCI performance for all completely paralyzed patients without any other means of communication. They showed that meaningful communication could not be achieved with a BCI for patients in CLIS, most of whom suffered from advanced ALS [6]. Notably, researchers had only used noninvasive BCIs up to that point. In 2011 the same group published two cases of CLIS with an invasive BCI that leverages a technique called electrocorticogram. For this technique, surgeons must implant electrodes directly on the surface of the exposed brain. Here again, no reliable and long-term communication of any kind was possible [7].

Meanwhile, another research team implanted a 96-microelectrode system into the motor cortices of several ALS patients and demonstrated fluent communication via a letter selection speller [8,9]. None of the ALS patients, however, were in CLIS; they all had other means of communication at their disposal. Even then, the speed of letter selection with the cellular BCI was highly satisfying.

Instrumental learning and complete paralysis

Birbaumer et al. [10] hypothesized several behavioral and physiological factors responsible for the lack of BCI control. One main determinant may be the extinction of goal-directed thinking. That is to say, patients in CLIS may no longer think in terms of producing voluntary actions to achieve particular outcomes. While an experiment using artificially paralyzed rats challenges this theory, the researchers failed to replicate their results [11]. Miller and collaborators intended to demonstrate that they could instrumentally train rats to control autonomic functions. A positive finding would imply that we can gain voluntary control of our inner organs, hormones, and physiological processes that are not usually under voluntary control. In contrast to the classical thinking of the physiology of the autonomic nervous system, Miller assumed that operant learning in the autonomous nervous system was possible. The group eliminated muscular responses by paralyzing rats and proceeded to reward the rats with intracranial positive self-stimulation for increasing and decreasing several autonomic functions such as heart rate, blood pressure, and blood volume. Despite initial success, these experiments could not be replicated by Miller and colleagues or any other laboratory since the time of publication in the 1980s. Thus we hypothesized that because patients in CLIS lose the association between output-oriented thinking and expected consequences, they can no longer learn instrumentally. Sensory imagery and auditory and tactile perception should remain intact, yet the absence of goal-directed physiology and behavior makes learning impossible.

We proposed that classical ("reflexive"), as opposed to instrumental ("operant"), learning and thinking remain intact in CLIS and in the curarized rat. In contrast to instrumental learning, classical conditioning does not depend on the production of a goal-reinforcement oriented response ("volition"), but rather depends on the passive association of a neutral warning conditioned stimulus (e.g., light) with an unconditioned stimulus (e.g., sight of food or shock). In support of this theory, Dworkin [12] found classical conditioning in the sciatic nerve of paralyzed rats who remained unresponsive to instrumental learning. We then developed a simple question and answer procedure to test the reflexive learning of brain responses to classify "yes" and "no" responses for patients in CLIS [13].

We measured the metabolic response of the brain using a technique called near-infrared spectroscopy (NIRS). NIRS is a noninvasive imaging technique which records changes in the concentration of oxyhemoglobin (HbO$_2$) and deoxyhemoglobin (Hb) in the cortex and serves as a proxy for neural activity. Emitters send photons inside the brain through the scalp, where these photons are absorbed by brain tissue. Some of these photons reach the upper layer of the brain tissue and some manage to scatter out of the brain, as presented in Fig. 4.1. The scattered photons are then measured by the detectors placed next to the emitters.

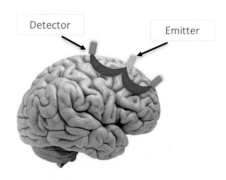

Figure 4.1 Example of the banana-shaped paths of light through the emitter–detector pair of NIRS device.

Self-regulation of brain metabolism

In earlier work [14], we showed that neurofeedback of the functional magnetic resonance imaging—derived blood oxygen level—dependent (BOLD) signal enables faster and more effortless learning of brain self-control, probably because the arterial and venous system of brain circulation sends feedback signals about its state (dilation, flow, etc.) to the brain. In contrast, neuroelectric processes have no receptor of their own activity and the brain is not informed about its neuroelectric changes. In addition, EEG is a much more complex neurophysiological process dependent upon many heterogeneous neuroanatomical systems and neuronal processes dampened and filtered by the head bone and skin. Such a variable response is much more difficult to classify as representing one single specific thought, namely "yes" and "no." As described previously, the lack of feedback from the neuroelectric process of neurons could indicate that learning based only on reinforcement, without sensory feedback information, is labile or nonexistent. We hypothesized that brain oxygenation and deoxygenation measured by functional NIRS (fNIRS) enables easier learning: a hypothesis confirmed by the results with CLIS patients [15]. Because patients answered "yes" and "no" questions correctly more than 70% of the time to questions with known answers (e.g., "Berlin is the capital of Germany"; "Berlin is the capital of France") without an obvious learning curve (the correct response rate remains stable over months), we assume that the classified physiological NIRS response reflects the mental "yes" or "no" answer present from the beginning of the BCI questioning ("all or none learning"). This, of course, is difficult to validate in completely paralyzed people, particularly for open questions to which only the patient knows the answer. The situation here is comparable to a lie detection scenario wherein the subject is notoriously uncooperative, and thus external validation by questioning the patient about the truth of the imagined answer remains impossible.

In addition to the papers by our laboratory, another group also used NIRS and reported similar success for "yes" and "no" communication in CLIS patients with

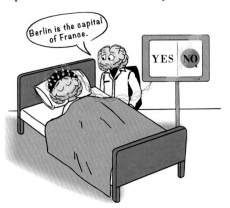

ALS [16]. However, no documentation of clinical or statistical data was provided. Even less gratifying is a publication by the owner of a BCI company [17]—using the EEG-BCI device manufactured by that company—which claimed that communication was achieved in two CLIS patients. Apart from the obvious conflict of interest, however, neither the clinical status of the patients nor quantitative or physiological results of the CLIS patients were made available.

Conclusions

Since the quality of life in locked-in patients with ALS who accept artificial respiration and are in family care is excellent—as reported in many publications in different countries and large samples—a functioning BCI system is vital so that such patients can continue to communicate when they reach the CLIS [18]. The difficulties in replicating noninvasive BCI procedures—in fNIRS and EEG alike—and the failure to communicate voluntarily by selecting letters or words from a BCI speller may necessitate an invasive approach that allows active communication in CLIS. With noninvasive BCI systems, we can only achieve passive communication with low precision and substantial errors when responding to simple "yes" or "no" questions. Thus, at present, implanted electrode systems allowing recording of neuronal firing and synaptic responses seems the only alternative to allow voluntary communication in complete paralysis.

Acknowledgments

The work was supported by the Deutsche Forschungsgemeinschaft (DFG), The European Union Horizon 2020: Luminous (Grant number: 686764) and the BMBF (Bundesministerium für Bildung und Forschung) CoMiCon (16SV7701), Wyss Center for Bio- and Neuroengineering, Geneva, Switzerland.

Additional readings

A successful textbook "Biological Psychology" that explores the relationships between biological processes and behavior: Birbaumer N, Schmidt RF. Biologische Psychologie. 7th ed. Heidelberg: Springer; 2010.

A popular style book arguing that the brain has almost limitless potentials and resembles a tabula rasa at birth—only a little is fixed, most of it is shaped: Birbaumer N. Your brain knows more than you think. Melbourne, London: Scribe; 2017.

Neurohype and the law: A cautionary tale

5

Stephen J. Morse

Many people think that neuroscience based on noninvasive brain imaging will transform how we view ourselves and our institutions, such as the law. Take, for example, the following editorial statement published in *The Economist* back in 2002.

> *Genetics may yet threaten privacy, kill autonomy, make society homogeneous and gut the concept of human nature. But neuroscience could do all of these things first [1].*

But neither genetics nor any other science that was predicted to revolutionize society and the law has had this effect. Neuroscience, which is simply the newest science on the block, is unlikely to produce the results *The Economist* fears, at least for the foreseeable future. At most, in the near to intermediate term, neuroscience may make modest contributions to legal policy and case adjudication. Nonetheless, there has been irrational exuberance about the potential contribution of neuroscience, a phenomenon I refer to as "Brain Overclaim Syndrome" [2,3]. Although I have prescribed a safe, effective, inexpensive treatment for this dire condition—"Cognitive Jurotherapy"—which simply requires learning the limitations of neuroscience and the conceptual relation between neuroscience and law, the disorder persists.

The reasons for neurohype are conceptual and empirical. Let's begin with the former. Law and neuroscience do not use the same language. Thus there will be problems of translation [4]. The law speaks the language of "folk psychology," the psychology we all use to explain our own behavior and the behavior of others in terms of mental states such as desires, beliefs, intentions, and reasons. For example, the explanation for why you are reading this chapter is, roughly, that you desire to learn something about the relevance of neuroscience to law, you believe that reading this

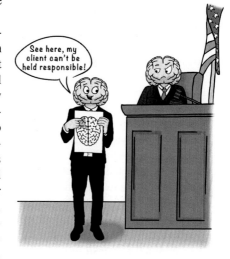

Casting Light on the Dark Side of Brain Imaging. DOI: https://doi.org/10.1016/B978-0-12-816179-1.00004-9

chapter might help achieve that goal, and thus you formed the intention to read it and you are now doing so. Legal rules are primarily about acts and mental states and are addressed to rational creatures who can be guided by rules.

In contrast, neuroscience is a mechanistic science that speaks the language of mechanism and in principle avoids folk-psychological concepts and discourse although neuroscientific articles are rife with dualistic discourse [5]. Neurons, neural networks, and the brain's connectome (see Chapter 23) do not have reasons. They have no aspirations, no sense of past, present, and future. They do not "do" things to each other. These are all properties of people. Brain images cannot tell us the reasons for a person's actions.

Can we bridge the chasm between the law's folk psychology and the mechanistic nature of neuroscience? This is a familiar question in the field of mental health law, but there is even greater dissonance when considering the relation of neuroscience to law. Psychiatry and psychology sometimes treat people as mechanisms, but also treat them as agents. Consequently, these disciplines are in part folk psychological, and the translation to law is easier than it is for neuroscience, which is purely mechanistic. Those claiming the relevance of neuroscience should always be able to explain precisely how neuroscientific findings, assuming that they are valid, are relevant to a legal issue.

Before turning to the current relation of neuroscience to law, let us quickly dispose of two "radical" challenges to law that neuroscience poses but that have had no legal purchase. The first is the belief that if determinism is true, which neuroscience allegedly proves, then responsibility is impossible. And yet, free will is not a criterion of any legal doctrine and is not even necessary to justify present doctrines of criminal responsibility [6]. Nonetheless, believing that no one is ever responsible for anything would upend criminal law and much of human interaction as we know it. No science can prove the truth of determinism, however, and there are good philosophical answers to the claim that determinism is incompatible with responsibility. "Neurodeterminism" is no more persuasive than all the other deterministic claims based on other sciences.

The more radical challenge is that neuroscience proves that we are just a pack of neurons or that we are simply victims of neuronal circumstances [7]. If this is true, we are less than simply not responsible; we are not agents who act for reasons. Mental states are just the foam on the neuronal wave. They exist but do nothing. This is a transformative claim, but on both conceptual and empirical grounds, there is simply no reason at present to believe that our mental states play no causal role in explaining behavior. Agency is secure.

The brain does enable the mind and action although we do not know how this occurs [8,9]. Facts we learn about brains in general or about a specific brain could in principle provide useful information about mental states and about human capacities in general and in specific cases. Some believe that this conclusion about the potential relevance of neuroscience is unwarranted. For the moment, let us bracket this pessimistic view and consider the relevance of neuroscience to resolving questions of criminal responsibility and other legal issues once the findings are properly translated into the law's folk-psychological framework.

Our question is whether some concededly valid neuroscience is legally relevant. Biological variables, including abnormal biological variables, do not per se answer any legal question because the law's criteria are behavioral—acts and mental states—and not biological. For example, even if a brain abnormality such as a tumor played a causal role in explaining a criminal defendant's behavior, it does not follow that a behavioral excusing condition, such as lack of rational or self-control capacity, was present. Any legal criterion must be established independently, and biological evidence must be translated into the law's folk-psychological criteria.

The advocate for using the data must be able to explain precisely how the neuro-data bear on the legal question in issue, such as whether a criminal defendant killed intentionally or whether the defendant was severely mentally disordered at the time of the crime. Does the tumor, for example, help confirm that the defendant's claim of mental disorder is true and how does it confirm it? If the evidence is not directly relevant, the advocate should be able to explain convincingly the chain of inference from the indirect evidence to the law's criteria.

Now let's turn to the empirical problems. The potential usefulness of neuro-science to law faces two major obstacles in addition to the problem of translation previously discussed. Despite the astonishing advances, behavioral neuroscience is not as advanced as we might hope. More directly relevant, there is a dearth of legally relevant studies. We shall discuss these two problems in order.

Space precludes detailed analysis of the general scientific difficulties, but the following considerations, discussed at length elsewhere [10], are important. Once again, we do not understand how the brain enables the mind and action. This does not present an insurmountable hurdle to good research, but it does hinder it. Most studies involve too few subjects to have sufficient statistical power and this casts doubt on the reproducibility of the results (see Chapter 12). Research design in behavioral neuroscience is particularly difficult and often makes clear inferences from results problematic. There are many response biases and artifacts (uncontrolled for variables) and more are constantly being identi-fied. Most of what we know is correlational and coarse, rather than causal and fine grained. The ability to generalize from laboratory findings to real world behavior—ecological validity—remains unclear. Performance on artificial tests in a scanner may not predict how people would behave in the rough and tumble world. The standard subjects of behavioral neuroscience studies are college stu-dents, who are hardly representative of the population generally or of, say, crim-inal offenders.

Finally, and perhaps most importantly for the law, there are few replications of studies. We cannot be sure that results are certain even if an individual study seems valid. There is a "replication crisis" in medicine and the social sciences and behav-ioral neuroscience is no exception (see Chapter 11). Lack of replications is particu-larly important for law (and medicine), which have such profound effects on people's lives. We don't want legal policy made or individual case outcomes affected by science that is quite uncertain. We certainly don't want a criminal defendant to be convicted and punished, or acquitted for that matter, based on the finding of one study.

None of these scientific concerns is surprising. Neuroimaging for general research is an infant science working on one of the hardest problems known to science, the relation of the brain to mental states, such as intentions, and to action. The proper methodologies are a work in progress. Many of these problems may be solved or substantially ameliorated in the future. For example, as the cost of imaging decreases, studies will be able to enroll more subjects. But many of these problems, such as the difficulties with inferences and the correlational nature of the research, will remain and present challenges.

The second major problem is that few studies have been addressed to normative legal questions, such as the nature of mental states that should ground culpability. In a recent review, an eminent neuroscientist and I reviewed all the behavioral neuroscience that might possibly be relevant to criminal law adjudication and policy. With the exception of studies of a few well-characterized medical conditions, such as epilepsy, that did *not* employ functional magnetic resonance imaging or other new techniques of noninvasive brain imaging, our review found virtually no solid neuroscience findings that were yet relevant [11]. Similar conclusions were reached after reviewing "brain reading" studies (e.g., "neural lie detection") [12] and neuroimaging research on addiction and criminal law [13].

There are some exceptions to this gloomy picture. Researchers have already carried out a few legally relevant, "proof-of-concept" studies about using neural variables to predict criminal reoffending [14] and to identify legally relevant mental states [15]. There are ongoing studies of potentially objective neural measures of how much subjective pain a subject is experiencing. This is of profound importance because the law's system of compensation in personal injury cases awards damages for pain and suffering based on mostly subjective assessment [16]. None of these studies or research projects is ready for practical use, but they do give a hint about the modest contributions that neuroscience may make to law in the near- or medium-term future.

Let us conclude with an observation that will always be germane even if neuroscience makes huge leaps forward. For the law, actions speak louder than images with very few exceptions. The law's criteria are behavioral—actions and mental states. If the finding of any test or measurement of behavior is contradicted by actual behavioral evidence, then we must believe the behavioral evidence because it is more direct and probative of the law's behavioral criteria. For example, if a criminal defendant behaves rationally in a wide variety of circumstances, the defendant is rational even if his or her brain appears structurally or functionally abnormal. In contrast, if the defendant is clearly psychotic, then a potentially legally relevant rationality problem exists even if his brain looks normal. We might think that neuroscience would be especially helpful in distinguishing the truth in "gray area" cases in which the behavioral evidence is unclear. For example, is the defendant simply very grandiose or actually delusional? But unfortunately the neuroscience helps us least when we need it the most, and if the behavior is clear, we don't need it at all.

In sum, despite major advances in behavioral neuroscience, the field has little to contribute to law at present. In the future, as the science develops, it will surely make contributions to legal policy and adjudication, but the law's underlying assumptions about human behavior and its concept of the person will remain largely unchanged.

Additional readings

Jones OD, Schall JD, Shen FX. Law and neuroscience. New York: Walters Kluwer; 2014 (the only legal casebook devoted to the field).

Pardo MS, Patterson D. Minds, brains, and law: the conceptual foundations of law and neuroscience. New York: Oxford University Press; 2013 (an introduction accessible to the interested lay reader).

Rosen, J. The brain on the stand. New York Times Magazine. March 11, 2007 (an excellent exposition of popular science writing).

Roth M. Philosophical foundations of neurolaw. Lanham, MD: Lexington Books; 2018. (technical but accessible introduction).

The brain in the classroom: The mindless appeal of neuroeducation

6

Gregory Donoghue

Since the 1990s scientists have promised a future where an increasingly sophisticated set of powerful brain-imaging tools would transform education as we know it. Nearly 30 years on, this future still hasn't arrived. In fact, neuroscience has yet to discover anything about education that good educators didn't already know. Consequently, educational practices remain largely unchanged since the emergence of educational neuroscience—or "neuroEd."

Not only is there no evidence of neuroscience knowledge impacting educational practice or learning outcomes, there is a growing number of academics making the compelling argument that neuroscience alone *can never* prescribe how teachers should teach [1−4]. Why not? Because, simply put, brains don't learn. People do. To see why the claims of neuroEd warrant such skepticism, and how commonly used brain scans are being misapplied, we need to understand precisely what learning is—and what it isn't.

Neuroscience takes it for granted that the brain causes—or at least mediates—all thoughts, emotions, physiological responses, and external behavior [5]. Before the emergence of neuroscience, learning was traditionally considered a "more or less permanent change in behavior as a result of experience" [6,7]. More recently however, neuroscience conceives of learning as a change in the brain—more specifically, in the number, strength and type of connections between neurons [8,9]. Brain scanning technology provides an imperfect window into these changes—allowing us to observe changes in the neuronal structure and operation that coincide with behavioral, physiological, emotional, and cognitive events in the whole person.

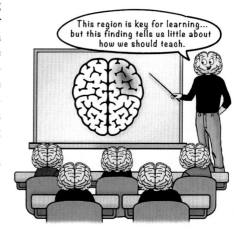

Casting Light on the Dark Side of Brain Imaging. DOI: https://doi.org/10.1016/B978-0-12-816179-1.00005-0

Observed differences in the brains of people who think, behave, emote, or believe in distinct ways are therefore unremarkable. That is to say, if Anne has a certain level of cognitive or physical ability, thinks a particular way, or believes a certain thing, it should come as no surprise that we would observe differences in her brain compared to that of Marie who has a different level of ability, or thinks or believes in different ways. In the educational context, we should find it equally unremarkable that a person with different capacities, abilities, or intelligence should produce different brain scans. After all, it is the brain that causes, or at least mediates, all of these outputs. Changes in those outputs must therefore correspond with changes in the brain—some of which are measurable by our current suite of neuroimaging tools.

While the literature is replete with examples of these scans—for example, the "brain on music" [10], or the traumatized brain [11]—such studies essentially draw correlations between a known event in the whole person (e.g., a stressful emotion), and an observable event in the person's brain (e.g., the activation of the amygdala). This does little more than confirm the presupposition that the brain causes or mediates all behavior, emotions, physiology, and cognition. Such studies do not directly identify the cause(s) of the phenomenon, and provide no insight into how to facilitate it. The pictures are alluring—but they are silent on the question that most interests educators and learning scientists: how do we systematically enhance the desirable outcomes of human learning?

Despite the seductive appeal of neuroscience, especially publications that feature alluring images of the human brain [12], neuroscience is yet to provide any evidence that would of itself decisively shape the professional practices of educators. The absence of a meaningful link between neuroscience and education has been demonstrated on empirical grounds [4]. In a sweeping review of the major neuroEd literature (covering some 565 articles), we were unable to find a *single neuroscientific study* whose conclusion pointed toward adopting any particular educational practice over another [13]. This finding was despite many claims that such evidence may, in the future, do so.

Skeptics have also argued against neuroEd on theoretical grounds [2,3,14] highlighting the logical fallacy of using evidence from one level of complexity (say, cellular neuroscience) and drawing prescriptive conclusions about practices at a higher level of complexity (such as a complex sociocultural context found in a classroom). Human learning is essentially a highly complex neurological process, while teaching occurs in a complex web of interpersonal, social, and cultural factors. Education therefore can be seen as even more complex than neuroscience—as it includes neuroscience *and* sociocultural factors. Drawing inferences directly from brain scans to education ignores the properties that emerge in that more complex level—properties that simply cannot be conceived, let alone predicted or confirmed at the lower level.

Consider this representative quotation from an international neuroEd conference that accompanied a brain scan of the intraparietal sulcus (IPS): "the IPS is really important in learning math. It shows that if I can get my students to think in the way that their brains want them to, I can really get them learning." While it is true that the IPS is involved in mathematics learning, it is nonsensical to suggest that brains *want* anything. *Wanting* is an emergent phenomenon that simply does not exist at the neurological level. Brains do not want. *People* want. Brain scans may be compelling and may even improve our understanding of the neural correlates of learning, but to suggest that they can prescribe how we teach and learn is currently a logical fallacy, pure, and simple. Brain scans capture the neural correlates of learning—not the learning itself. The map is not the territory.

To see this fallacy illustrated, we need look no further than a recent, high-quality electroencephalogram study [15]. The authors produced a compelling brain-scan image of the "brain on growth mind-set" (where the person believes that effort can improve one's ability) compared to a "brain on fixed mind-set" (where the person believes that their ability is unchangeable).

The authors of this study validly concluded that there were measurable differences between the brain scans of people with a "growth mind-set" and those with a "fixed mind-set." More specifically, they stated that "people who think they can learn ... have different brain reactions" [16] and that "... brain activity and cognitive control can be altered after reading a short article ... regarding abilities" [17]. While these conclusions may be reasonable, they do not follow the evidence provided by the brain scans. The tendency to make overly broad conclusions on this type of evidence is very common in the neuroEd field. For example, one commercial enterprise used this study to declare that:

> ... when we make a mistake, synapses fire. A synapse is an electrical signal that moves between parts of the brain when learning occurs... [this] is hugely important for math teachers and parents, as it tells us that making a mistake is a very good thing. Mistakes are not only opportunities for learning, as students consider the mistakes, but also times when our brains grow [18].

Such a claim is a representative example of going way beyond the evidence while attempting to derive greater credibility from citing a neuroscientific source, complete with alluring brain-scan images [12]. Others claimed that this evidence "could help in training people to believe that they can work harder and learn more, by showing how their brain is reacting to mistakes" [16]. While this type of neurological evidence may generate hypotheses about what may happen in the classroom, it does not allow for such broad conclusions. In fact, the only evidence that can confirm best educational practices must be drawn from that educational context—not from a brain scan.

This is not to say that neuroscience has no role in educational research—it does, just not a prescriptive role. Instead, integrating neuroscience into education requires careful translation between the layers of complexity. A good example of how neuroscience can inform education has been demonstrated by the Science of Learning Research Centre [19]. Their PEN (Pyschology Education Neuroscience) principles comprise 12 core tenets in learning and teaching that are supported by evidence from each of the three layers of complexity most directly implicated in the learning process. These are good examples of how prescriptive conclusions about what works in education are ultimately based on evidence from that educational context, while evidence from the two layers of lower complexity are drawn upon to confirm, explain, conceptualize, and generate hypotheses.

Until we more fully understand the neurological processes involved in learning, and we have developed nonpedagogical tools that can directly change brains in predictable and precise ways—such as electrical or magnetic stimulation techniques (see Chapter 18)—human learning will continue to be mediated behaviorally, experientially, and pedagogically. Until then, neuroscience cannot prescribe educational practices.

The human brain is one of the most complex structures in the universe, and learning about it is a highly desirable pursuit. Educators may even find it worth their while to study the brain—if only to enable more informed decisions about brain-based products and programs. Brain scans will continue to inform, conceptualize, explain, and theorize—but they will never prescribe how educators best teach, or how students best learn. Human learning will continue to be enhanced by educators who for thousands of years have been dedicated to their craft of teaching people, not brains.

Additional reading

Horvath, J.C. & Donoghue, G.M. So much talk about the 'the brain' in education is meaningless. The conversation 2015. <http://theconversation.com/so-much-talk-about-the-brain-in-education-is-meaningless-47102>.

Section II

What are we measuring?

Brain waves: How to decipher the cacophony

7

Suresh Muthukumaraswamy

Recording electrical signals from the surface of our head is almost too easy. The hard part is distinguishing what part of the signal comes from the brain and what part from muscle activity. Facial musculature, eye movements, blinks, and even the beating of the heart can contaminate electrical recordings of the brain with signals orders of magnitude larger than those produced by the brain. We can easily lose brain signals in the cacophony of these artifacts. Indeed, almost every popular representation of brain waves overlooks this issue. While scientists can easily discard periods of data where these large artifacts occur, the smaller artifacts tend to be more pernicious. They often escape the notice of investigators and their artifact detection algorithms. In this chapter, we explore what brain waves are, how scientists can misread their meaning, and how to judiciously interpret brain data.

So, what are brain waves and how do we measure them? In essence, brain waves are the accumulation of electrical activity from millions of brain cells. When one brain cell sends information to another, they use chemical transmitters that cause the receiving cell to generate small electrical potentials. Single brain cells produce tiny potentials, but the brain has evolved so that tens of thousands of brain cells will "fire" nearly simultaneously. Moreover, the most common type of cell in the cerebral cortex, the pyramidal cell (so named because of their shape), tends to share the same orientation in respect to the surface of the brain. With this combination of temporal synchrony and geometric alignment, the electrical potentials of brain cells summate and become large enough to detect on the scalp surface with electrodes. When combined with appropriate amplifiers and displays, this summation allows scientists to record the well-known electroencephalogram (EEG).

Following the basic laws of physics, every electrical potential will have a corresponding set of magnetic fields. Using specialized detectors and a magnetically shielded room, scientists can measure these tiny magnetic fields with a magnetoencephalogram (MEG). These instruments are much more difficult to engineer than the simple electrodes used for EEG. As such, MEG devices are less common, less well-known, and much more expensive than EEG (costing millions as opposed to thousands of dollars). While there are subtle differences between the signals these techniques record, broadly speaking, both techniques measure the summated activity of pyramidal cells and we will refer to them together as M/EEG.

Compared with other types of brain imaging, M/EEG can be particularly satisfying for scientists who study the human brain. Unlike functional magnetic resonance

Casting Light on the Dark Side of Brain Imaging. DOI: https://doi.org/10.1016/B978-0-12-816179-1.00006-2

imaging (fMRI), which measures a blood signal that lags behind brain activity by 4−6 seconds, M/EEG records brain activity *directly* and can be seen virtually in real time on a computer monitor (and in former times drawn directly onto paper sheets). In most healthy participants, after setting up EEG electrodes and amplifiers, one can simply ask participants to relax and close their eyes, which will reliably generate large "alpha" waves, with a frequency of around 10 Hz, from the posterior areas of the brain. But the production of other brain waves remains less well understood.

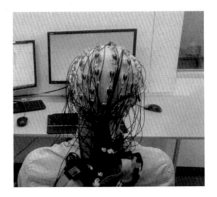

Figure 7.1 A modern EEG system with 64 electrodes. Some systems use up to 256 electrodes.

For example, scientists continue to debate the significance of "gamma waves," which have a frequency range of about 30−90 Hz. In the 1990s two pioneering experiments used electrodes directly implanted in the visual cortices of cats and detected gamma waves in response to visual stimuli [1]. Researchers subsequently speculated that these gamma waves may be a neural correlate of consciousness. This speculation caused great excitement in the scientific community, and served to focus the attention of many M/EEG scientists into the higher frequency bands of the M/EEG.

Up until that time, most M/EEG scientists had generally focused on lower frequency waves such as delta (1−4 Hz), theta (4−8 Hz), alpha (8−13 Hz), and beta (13−30 Hz), while filtering out higher frequencies. These frequencies were filtered in order to remove potential muscle contamination, which is most heavily concentrated in

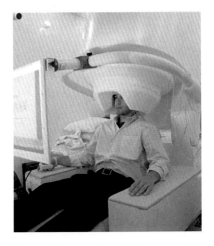

Figure 7.2 A modern MEG system with 275 channels. The detectors sit inside the "hairdryer", just a few centimeters from the head of the volunteer, and are bathed in liquid helium at -269°C.

the 20−200 Hz range, from the data. Unfortunately, this frequency band of muscle activity exactly overlaps with the gamma-band! Subsequent to the findings in cats, numerous studies used EEG to look at "gamma" responses to visual stimuli in humans. The responses looked strikingly similar to those observed in cats. Only later did further research show that in many cases, these "gamma" responses were in fact artifacts caused by tiny eye movements, called microsaccades, which occur automatically in response to the stimuli [2].

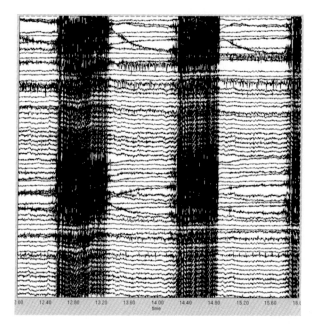

Figure 7.3 Some nasty EEG data recorded using the EEG setup shown earlier. I asked the volunteer to clench their jaw every few seconds. There is quite a bit of muscle activity even in the quieter periods and a few electrodes are drifting.

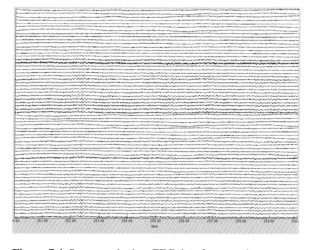

Figure 7.4 Some much nicer EEG data from a volunteer relaxed with their eyes open. Small alpha waves can be seen.

In a similar vein, a beautiful series of studies from a research group in Australia has shown that even the so-called clean EEG data, recorded from participants at rest, can be quite heavily contaminated by background muscle activity [3]. To demonstrate this point the scientists compared the EEG activity of volunteers under normal conditions against that obtained under a condition of conscious full body paralysis. Full body paralysis was achieved by injecting the paralyzing agent cisatracurium, whose grandparent molecule curare was used in the blow darts of indigenous South American tribes to asphyxiate their prey. The paralysis condition eliminates all muscle activity, requiring ventilators for respiratory support and showed a massive reduction in "gamma" activity in the EEG of the volunteers. The implication being that much of the extra "gamma" activity seen in the normal EEG is actually background muscle noise, absent during paralysis.

Ask yourself for a second, would you volunteer to be completely paralyzed, but conscious in such an experiment? Thanks to these brave volunteers (who were also members of the research team!) we learned some valuable lessons about M/EEG. The lessons were not that gamma activity cannot be recorded in the M/EEG—indeed, my personal research group regularly publishes work looking at gamma activity in M/EEG. Quite the contrary the point here is that scrupulous self-criticism of data, careful experimentation, thorough peer-review and scientific discussion is *necessary* to make progress. While these errors are unfortunate, and some continue to occur, the quality of data and analysis is undoubtedly improving. Over time the scientific literature seems to self-correct—but it may take a few years!

When we do manage to isolate brain activity from the M/EEG signal, what can we learn from these squiggly traces? Why does an activated cortex amplify gamma waves (30−90 Hz) but suppress alpha waves (8−13 Hz)? Why do theta waves (4−8 Hz) emerge during memory tasks but also during the transition to sleep? For these questions, taking a historical perspective helps. The EEG is the oldest technique we have for measuring brain function with German psychiatrist Hans Berger reporting the first EEG recordings in 1929. From a sociocultural perspective, this longer history makes the field of EEG significantly different to that of fMRI—the other mainstay of functional brain imaging which was first reported in 1990. How so you might ask? Well to be blunt, many of the pioneers who developed the first techniques, tools, and studies using fMRI are still with us, whereas generations of M/EEG scientists have long since passed on. For the modern neuroscientist like myself to look back at these early, often forgotten, but seminal EEG studies (1930−60) are fascinating. For example, in 1931 Berger speculated that alpha activity is associated with psychophysical processes while beta activity is associated with metabolic processes of cortical tissues [4]. Both these hypotheses are strikingly similar to ideas that exist today with regards to the role of alpha rhythms in attention and the relation of beta oscillations to fMRI activations. This suggests somewhat embarrassingly that our fundamental theoretical understanding of the function of these rhythms has not come very far in the last 80 years! Certainly a greater understanding of what has gone before will aid the modern scientist to avoid repeating previous theories without proper historical context but will also help us to avoid repeating past mistakes.

It remains a challenge to decipher exactly what the M/EEG signal represents, remembering that it takes the collective and synchronized activity of tens of thousands of neurons and millions of synapses (the connections between neuron) to produce sufficient activity for us to record at the scalp. Not only that, but multiple cell types are involved and they use diverse chemical transmitters to communicate with each other. The mind really boggles at the complexity and numbers involved. While difficult for a human to grasp, advances in computing technology now allow us to generate increasingly sophisticated computational models of how this underlying circuitry might work. By continuing to perform well controlled M/EEG experiments, using careful data analysis, and combining these advances with improving computational models of how M/EEG signals are generated, we have a good opportunity to understand the behavior of the M/EEG. Many of the major pitfalls in discriminating M/EEG signals from artifact sources have now been worked out and readers of M/EEG studies can have much greater confidence in the results than ever before. Hopefully the insights into brain activity that M/EEG provides will give us understanding into not only how the brain works, but also be useful in helping the diagnosis and treatments of those patients who suffer from neurological and psychiatric disorders.

Additional readings

A detailed examination of electrophysiological signals and their meaning: Buzsaki G. Rhythms of the brain. Oxford University Press; 2006.

A freely available academic review of EEG and muscle activity: Muthukumaraswamy S. High-frequency brain activity and muscle artifacts in MEG/EEG: a review and recommendations. Front Hum Neurosci 2013;7:138.

Scholarpedia and Wikipedia are quite useful to find out more about M/EEG and the nature of brain activity, <http://www.scholarpedia.org/article/Electroencephalogram>, <https://en.wikipedia.org/wiki/Gamma_wave>, <https://en.wikipedia.org/wiki/Neural_oscillation>.

On the relationship between functional MRI signals and neuronal activity

8

Amir Shmuel

Can you picture the last image of brain activity you saw? Perhaps it was in a magazine or online article. Chances are, those maps were derived from data collected with functional magnetic resonance imaging (fMRI) and probably looked similar to Fig. 8.1. Like other functional brain imaging techniques, researchers use fMRI to estimate changes in the brain activity of humans in health and disease [1−3].

The most commonly used fMRI method measures changes in the oxygen content of blood [4]. More specifically, this procedure records signals that track increases and decreases in the local content of deoxyhemoglobin (deoxyHb)—a molecule found in deoxygenated blood. Following increases in neuronal activity in a circumscribed brain region, the blood supply to that region will increase in order to replenish the oxygen and glucose that were consumed to support the elevated neuronal activity. The relative increase in blood flow is greater than the rise in oxygen consumption [5−6]. This process causes a drop of deoxyHb content in the local capillaries, venules, and draining veins, which increases the magnitude of the fMRI blood oxygenation signal [7]. This measure is known as the blood oxygen level−dependent (BOLD) signal and is often mapped onto structural images of the brain to depict brain activity under different circumstances or between groups of individuals (as shown in Fig. 8.1). Another fMRI methods, which is becoming popular, estimates changes in the amount of blood within a given area of brain tissue—known as cerebral blood volume (CBV) [8].

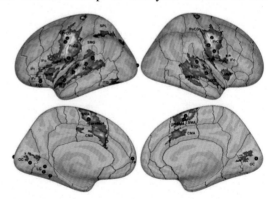

Figure 8.1 Brain activity while producing single words or pseudo-words plotted on inflated cortical surfaces.

Adapted from Guenther, Frank H., Neural Control of Speech, Figure 2.14, p. 60, © 2016 Massachusetts Institute of Technology, by permission of The MIT Press.

Casting Light on the Dark Side of Brain Imaging. DOI: https://doi.org/10.1016/B978-0-12-816179-1.00007-4

Nonneuroscientists often overlook an important reality of fMRI—neither the BOLD signal nor the CBV method is a direct measure of neuronal activity. Instead, fMRI is used to infer changes in neuronal activity based on local changes in metabolism and blood flow. Such changes have been shown experimentally to accompany changes in neuronal activity, but the relationship is not necessarily one to one. Below are five points to help unpack the relationship between neuronal activity and fMRI signals.

1. *As neuronal activity increases, so do fMRI signals*

While researchers continue to hash out the details of the relationship between fMRI signals and local neural activity, it is well established that increases in metabolism and blood flow measured with fMRI are associated with increases in neural activity. Many studies go further and demonstrate a proportional relationship between these two measures. For example, when researchers stimulate the cerebellum of a rat, blood flow and neuronal activity amplify proportionally [9]. When presenting visual stimuli to individuals, the blood oxygenation in parts of their cortex increase proportionally to the corresponding increases in neuronal activity [10,11]. Similarly the rate of oxygen consumption is proportional to increases in neuronal activity [12]. This relationship, however, is not always proportional. For example, experiments show that as the intensity of a stimulus increases, blood flow continues to rise whereas neuronal responses plateau [13−15].

Neurons use two forms of related electrochemical activity to communicate: action potentials and synaptic activity. Action potentials form an all-or-none signal that propagates from the cell body of a neuron to its output processes, namely the axons. Action potentials that reach axon terminals induce a change in the voltage of connected neurons. This change in voltage is called synaptic activity. The BOLD signal appears to be related to the local synaptic activity, which is caused by local neuronal activity as well as other inputs from more distant parts of the brain. Under most experimental conditions the BOLD response is similarly related to action potentials. However, in cases where we can dissociate synaptic activity from action potentials, the BOLD response seems to more closely reflect local synaptic activity [11,16].

2. *fMRI cannot detect sparse neuronal activity*

Electrodes inserted directly into the brain are much better than fMRI at detecting neuronal activity [11]. Thus fMRI can lead to "false negatives" when it sometimes statistically rejects low-amplitude neuronal responses that are both detectable with electrodes and in reality statistically significant. Averaging fMRI responses over multiple imaging sessions can reduce noise and allow researchers to correctly classify more brain regions as activated [17].

3. *Compared to the millisecond and micrometric resolution of neuronal activity, fMRI has a temporal precision in the order of seconds and a spatial precision down to about 1 mm [3]*

In the temporal domain the BOLD response appears as a lagged, sluggish, smoothed version of the neuronal response (Fig. 8.2). The difference between the signals manifests because changes in blood flow occur on a slower timescale than changes in electrophysiological activity. While the electrophysiological response may take place within milliseconds or tens of milliseconds following sensory stimuli, the blood oxygenation response transpires within hundreds of milliseconds to seconds. Typically, we observe the peak blood flow and blood oxygenation 5–6 seconds after the onset of a stimulus. Hence, a second stimulus can arrive while a brain region's vascular activity is still developing in response to an initial neuronal event.

The spatial specificity of fMRI signals depends on the fMRI method, the strength of the magnetic field, and which aspect of the vasculature is being probed (e.g., capillaries, venules, or veins). The spatial spread of the combined neuronal and BOLD response in the human visual area (V1) is about 3.5 mm at a low magnetic field (1.5 T [18]) and less than 2 mm at a high magnetic field (7 T [19]). The net spatial spread of blood oxygenation responses at 7 T relative to the

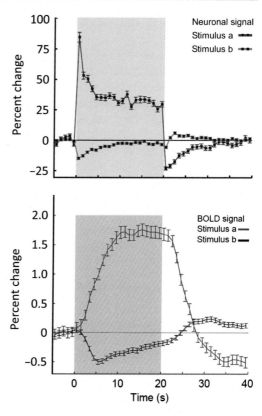

Figure 8.2 Upper panel: time course (mean ± SEM) of the neuronal activity in the visual cortex in response to rotating checkerboard stimuli. Lower panel: time course (mean ± SEM) of the blood oxygenation fMRI response sampled from a region in the visual cortex, activated by the same rotating checkerboard stimuli. Adapted from Shmuel et al., 2006, *Nature Neuroscience*, 9(4): 569–577.

site of increased neuronal activity has been estimated as ~1.0 mm [20].

Recent studies in animals [21] and humans [22] have demonstrated that fMRI based on estimating CBV (rather than the BOLD signal) is spatially specific to the site of increased neuronal activity. In other words, it reflects the spatial pattern of increased neuronal activity at high fidelity. It may approach the level of spatial specificity required for imaging responses of the six layers of the cerebral cortex [21,22].

4. *Neuronal activity and fMRI signals are associated in the resting brain*

Studies conducted over the past two decades have demonstrated that human brain activity, as measured by fMRI, occurs in a highly organized fashion even when individuals are not exposed to stimuli or given a task. These resting-state fluctuations are correlated over large parts of the human brain, a phenomenon termed "functional connectivity," and are consistent between subjects [23] (see Chapter 23 for more details). Resting-state fMRI may be useful for early detection of neurological and psychiatric conditions, because the organization of brain activity, as measurable with fMRI, is modified early on in the progression of such conditions. To correctly interpret fMRI recorded in the resting state, it is important to study the corresponding relationship between the fMRI signal and the underlying neuronal activity.

Since neuronal activity in the resting state is spontaneous, with no stimuli or task, researchers must simultaneously record both fMRI and neuronal activity to understand their relationship in the resting state. Using simultaneous fMRI and neurophysiological recordings, we demonstrated an association between the slow fluctuations in fMRI signals and concurrent fluctuations in the underlying local neuronal activity [24]. We consistently identified these associations when the neuronal signal consisted of either variations in synaptic activity [24,25] or the rate of action potentials [24].

5. *In some instances, neuronal activity and fMRI responses dissociate*

The previous sections focused on cases that reported metabolic and blood flow responses that corresponded to changes in neurophysiological activity. A few studies reported cases in which these signals dissociated. For example, one study measured both the BOLD signal and electrophysiology of monkeys in a paradigm where a visual stimulus may become subjectively invisible [26]. All brain signals were associated when the stimulus was subjectively visible. However, when the stimulus became subjectively invisible, only the BOLD signal and the slow synaptic activity showed decreases, whereas the action potentials and fast changing synaptic activity remained unaffected.

While these researchers did observe changes in bands of lower frequencies electrophysiological activity that corresponded to the changes in BOLD signal, other researchers found evidence of a complete divergence of blood flow and neurophysiological signals [27]. Using an optical imaging technique that measures CBV and blood oxygenation, these researchers found two distinct components to the hemodynamic signal in the primary visual cortex of awake monkeys (V1). One component was reliably predictable from neuronal responses generated by visual input. The other component, of almost comparable strength, was reported as an unknown signal that entrains to the task structure independently of the visual input or of standard neural predictors of changes in blood flow.

Note that both studies [26,27] pursued their measurements in alert animals, in contrast to the majority of other studies of neurovascular coupling that used anesthetized animals. This indicates that neurovascular coupling may be modified in the alert state, possibly via the action of neuromodulators that depend on the behavioral state. This finding adds to the complexity of the interplay between neurophysiological signals and blood flow responses, which surely will be addressed in future studies.

What is functional magnetic resonance imaging most useful for?

fMRI is very useful for estimating the regions of the brain that respond to sensory stimuli or to tasks. fMRI can also address questions on the relative amplitude of responses to two or more conditions, as long as the comparison is done with data from the exact same region of the brain. In addition, fMRI is useful for detecting regions of the brain which show functional connectivity, that is, their fMRI-based activities are synchronized during task or spontaneous activity (resting state). fMRI cannot directly address questions on neuronal activity; it only infers changes in neuronal activity based on hemodynamic and metabolic responses. Lastly, fMRI cannot address questions on changes in neuronal activity at a fine temporal scale; it can only infer change in neuronal activity at the temporal scale of 2−3 seconds or longer.

Conclusion

fMRI records signals based on increased metabolism and blood flow in response to increased activity of the brain. Under specific paradigms or brain states, the fMRI response and the local neuronal activity may dissociate. However, in the vast majority of cases, the fMRI response in a voxel correlates with the overall neuronal activity within the voxel.

Additional readings

Bakker A. Basics of fMRI − principles and methods of neuroimaging. <https://www.coursera.org/lecture/neuroscience-neuroimaging/basics-of-fmri-mC6Om>. The link directs to a video, presented by Dr. Arnold Bakker from Johns Hopkins Department of Psychiatry. The video is part of the coursera course on "Fundamental Neuroscience for Neuroimaging".

Yuhas D. What's a voxel and what can it tell us? A primer on fMRI. Scientific American blog; 2012. <https://blogs.scientificamerican.com/observations/whats-a-voxel-and-what-can-it-tell-us-a-primer-on-fmri/>.

MRI artifacts in psychiatry: Head motion, breathing, and other systematic confounds

Robert T. Thibault and Amir Raz

To better understand psychiatric conditions, we rarely look at the brains of cadavers any more, but that was common practice some hundred years ago. Today, magnetic resonance imaging (MRI) and functional MRI (fMRI), to give one example, permit structural and functional investigation of the biology of psychiatric conditions in the living human brain. And yet, many subtle pitfalls linger when imaging the neural infrastructure, let alone neural activity, in search of higher brain functions.

Not only does the popular science press burst at the seams with images of scanned brains, leading psychiatry journals now regularly include findings from brain imaging assays. A typical experiment may draw on about two dozen people from one group, often individuals diagnosed with a mental disorder, and compare these patients to a comparably sized group of controls. Unfortunately, these findings tell us considerably less than most readers appreciate. Why? Mostly because of inadequate statistical power (see Chapter 12) and systematic confounds. For example, patients and controls often differ with respect to traits that alter brain data (e.g., head motion in the scanner) without necessarily affecting the underlying neural activity. Such confounds pervade findings from both structural and functional brain imaging research.

With structural brain imaging, we often hear largely accepted, but nonetheless questionable, statements such as "anxiety alters amygdala volume," "depression shrinks hippocampus and cingulate cortex," and "schizophrenia eats away at cortical matter." While debate wages on, many researchers acquiesce to the notion that structural brain changes are a primary characteristic of psychiatric disorders [1]. Some researchers even claim that nonpathological behaviors, such as watching porn [2], alter the structure of our brain. Thus we apply diagnostic terms, such as "cortical thinning," "atrophy," "tissue loss," and "abnormal connectivity," and we assume that these are insights into the underlying nature of these conditions [3].

We'd like to make sure you fully understand our point: we don't challenge the findings that these studies report; instead, we contest the jargon filled, authoritative mode, which colors their seemingly conclusive claims. Such presentations conceal

Casting Light on the Dark Side of Brain Imaging. DOI: https://doi.org/10.1016/B978-0-12-816179-1.00008-6

a largely ignored, inconvenient truth: MRI scarcely allows us to make firm inferences about the neurobiology of mental disorders.

To begin to understand why, remind yourself what this imaging technique really measures. MRI does not directly assess brain structure (see Chapter 8). Rather, it measures the properties of hydrogen atoms and depends on the magnetic properties of the microenvironment surrounding the tissue. In other words, MR signals are susceptible to many physical–chemical phenomena possibly unrelated to the number (or structure) of cells in tissue.

When MRI scans emerge as evidence for a linkage between a given psychiatric condition and a certain pathology of brain structures, we must consider alternative, nonanatomical explanations. For example, some factors that influence MR signals include history of smoking, alcohol, cannabis/psychedelic drugs, exercise, body weight, lipid levels, ongoing stress, and medication.

Slight head motion during a scan can wield a substantial impact on MRI findings. So "professional" control participants—that is, individuals who partake in multiple MRI experiments as paid volunteers—would likely have the advantage of keeping more still, compared to the uninitiated. Now imagine individuals diagnosed with a psychiatric disorder, their symptoms managed by medication, entering an MRI machine for the first time and asked to lie motionless for extended periods of time. Is it possible the image from the patient brain exhibits "cortical volume and thickness reduction," or was the difference a function of how the patient subtly *moved* compared to a control participant?

To further illustrate this point, consider the "excessive tissue loss" in the hippocampus observed via MRI in schizophrenic patients. If this observation were a result of abnormalities in the neurobiology, then evidence of such tissue loss should be apparent upon a postmortem examination. Alas, more than a hundred years of postmortem studies have scantily confirmed this MRI-based result [3].

In fMRI experiments, we usually see "activation" studies, where participants perform a particular task, and "resting-state" studies where participants lie passively in the scanner without any specific cognitive goal. Over a thousand peer-review scientific reports on fMRI are published each year, and yet most of these articles neglect to mention common confounds—often the very same ones that plague structural MRI findings. While fMRI has improved dramatically since its inception in 1992, researchers still fall into the same traps of oversight and omission when comparing patients to healthy controls.

Within activation studies, rigorous experimental designs can offset many a confound. However, resting-state fMRI studies, where participants go through a scan without a specific task, pose a conundrum because participants experience the scanning process very differently, thereby exerting a dramatic impact on fMRI data. To demonstrate why many resting-state fMRI findings are likely spurious, one research group looked at a dataset of 500 brain scans, all taken from healthy controls, and tested every permutation of 20 brains compared to 20 other brains [4]. They found significant differences between the two groups of brains in up to 70% of cases. Moreover, they used the default setting in many statistical packages, which assumes that fMRI data follow a certain distribution, although that's frequently untrue. In other words, some "standard methods" of analysis that rest on unreliable assumption can easily produce false positives. Thus we must remain wary of the default statistical methods as we attempt to sort out results: from the robust to the flimsy.

Rather than direct neural activity, fMRI measures the content of oxygen in the blood circulating throughout the brain (the blood oxygen level dependent (BOLD) signal). If we hold our breath during a scan, we can drive a 3%−6% change in the BOLD signal [5−7]. Meanwhile, most fMRI studies find differences of less than 1% between experimental groups. Moreover, not just holding the breath, but subtle variations in respiratory rate and depth—patterns

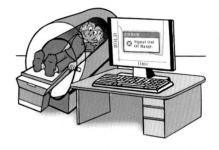

that occur naturally over time—can also markedly sway the BOLD signal [8,9]. Can you imagine breathing differences when you cram anxious patients into an MRI scanner and compare them to healthy controls? Is it possible that these two groups would breathe differently? Don't hold your breath for the correct answer.

Two "hot" regions in brain imaging research—the anterior cingulate and the insula—are particularly susceptible to respiratory artifacts. Could their fame rely on such inhale−exhale confounds? Perhaps, but we would need further studies to confirm. With appropriate methodology, including a chest belt and some statistical modeling, we can control for and rule out a substantial portion of this potential artifact. And yet, not all neuroimagers pursue this direction.

Now consider imaging the brains of expert meditators, say Buddhist monks who have been practicing their contemplative tradition for decades. If we compared their resting state to that of naïve controls, would you not expect the monks to be thinking about very different things? Would you not suppose that they breathe differently? Lining up a large sample of expert meditators would make for a tall order, so a small group would have to do and the possibility of a false positive would accordingly become more prominent, especially if we draw on default statistical tests. To properly evaluate fMRI resting-state findings, we would need to account, at the very least, for the sample size and what participants were pondering, whether the researchers had regressed out distortion from breathing, and whether they used appropriate stats.

The status of neuroimaging research in psychiatry seems tenuous. On the one hand, (f)MRI remains an important tool for understanding the psychopathology and pathobiology of mental disorders. On the other hand, to make further advances, researchers ought to keep in mind the caveats we have highlighted herein, and which remain heretofore largely unaddressed. Toward this end, clinicians and researchers stand to benefit from designing and interpreting experiments that account for such potential artifacts. We would do well to critically rethink the inferences we sometimes draw from (f)MRI studies of mental health.

Additional readings

The experiment showing a high rate of false-positive in certain types of fMRI studies: Eklund A, Nichols TE, Knutsson H. Cluster failure: why fMRI inferences for spatial extent have inflated false-positive rates. Proc Natl Acad Sci USA 2016;113(7900−7905):201602413. Available from: https://doi.org/10.1073/pnas.1602413113.

A more in depth discussion on artifacts in (f)MRI, and inspiration for this chapter: Weinberger DR, Radulescu E. Finding the elusive psychiatric "lesion" with 21st-century neuroanatomy: a note of caution. Am J Psychiatry 2016;173(1):27−33. Available from: https://doi.org/10.1176/appi.ajp.2015.15060753.

When the brain lies: Body posture alters neural activity

10

Robert T. Thibault

Imagine if researchers were up front about what awaits the subject of a typical brain imaging session: "Welcome to the lab, please lie down and keep your head absolutely still. We'll slide you into this tube here and be back in an hour. These earbuds will help block out any sudden screeches and thumps—of which there will be plenty. Good luck."

Now, for many clinical and research purposes, this situation poses only negligible problems. But what if we aim to understand the brain processes of everyday human functioning? How likely is it that a typical person will respond to the contrived environment of a magnetic resonance imaging (MRI) session in a similar manner as they would to a more familiar, ecological context? For researchers looking to model brain processes associated with day-to-day activity, such questions point toward a serious concern—we must treat the brain not as a jumble of neurons in a vat, but as a component of a body that interacts with its environment.

Lying motionless in a cramped tube or sitting alone in a silent and dimly lit room remains far from a run-of-the-mill afternoon. And yet, much of our knowledge of the functioning human brain stems from such settings. If we closely examine the constraints that neuro-imaging experiments impose, we can start to understand how these experimental settings affect us. One oft-overlooked source of discrepancy between experimental and everyday contexts—namely, body posture—not only changes the way our neurons fire, but also alters the way we feel pain, breathe, think, and even see. It turns out that whether participants sit, stand, or lie down can dramatically impact the results of a brain imaging study.

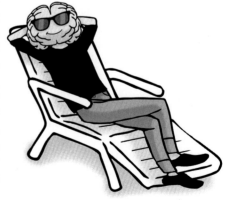

Casting Light on the Dark Side of Brain Imaging. DOI: https://doi.org/10.1016/B978-0-12-816179-1.00009-8

To better appreciate how brain imaging environments alter our mental and physical states, we must first examine what these environments look like. Today, most functional neuroimaging—that is to say, measures of brain function rather than brain structure—record either electromagnetic signals or the level of oxygen in the blood circulating throughout the brain. The physical constraints vary with the method. For example, in a typical electroencephalography (EEG) experiment (see Chapter 7), participants sit alone in an eerily quiet room and stare at a computer screen for extended periods of time. In a standard functional MRI (fMRI) experiment (see Chapter 8), participants lie motionless in a narrow cylinder while loud hums and thumps revolve around their head for up to an hour. While functional neuroimaging generally draws on these two technologies, researchers sometimes opt for other techniques such as magnetoencephalography (MEG) and functional near infrared spectroscopy (fNIRS).

Each imaging modality permits a subset of body positions. Participants can wear EEG and fNIRS caps throughout a wide range of postures and, with proper equipment, can move and interact with their environment; MEG machines often restrict participants to an adjustable seat that can adopt any position between an upright chair and a horizontal bench; and most fMRI options constrain participants to horizontal positions. Compared to portable technologies (EEG and fNIRS) the large and static imaging devices (fMRI and MEG) permit fewer postures, yet provide higher quality data. These intrinsic differences make certain imaging modalities more advantageous for specific applications and research questions but less so for others. For example, the postural constraints of most MRI scanners would make fMRI a good way to explore the resting brain, but less ideal to study the brain of a motorist at the wheel.

The truth, which many studies avoid addressing directly, is that the imaging environment, by restricting the range of available postures, can alter the very mental phenomena researchers aim to study. Take the simple difference between upright and lying subjects. Not only do we perform motor tasks better when sitting upright but we also smell certain odors better, feel pain more intensely, and asses our visual field differently [1−4]. Sitting amplifies our anxiety, increases motivation, hinders conflicting thoughts, and improves nonverbal intelligence compared to lying down [4,5]. On the flip side, whereas upright postures can improve our selective attention [6], they can compromise performance on problems requiring a burst of insight [7].

Sitting and standing also affect physiology and increase our heart rate, respiratory volume, oxygen consumption, core body temperature, and the release of a stress hormone known as cortisol [8−11]. Body posture further regulates the volume and flow of blood throughout the brain [12]. Notably, these processes represent the very signal that fMRI measures: blood-oxygen concentrations—not, as is often presumed, neural activity itself (see Chapter 8). Thus posture can influence the fMRI signal via mechanisms independent of the activity of neurons [13].

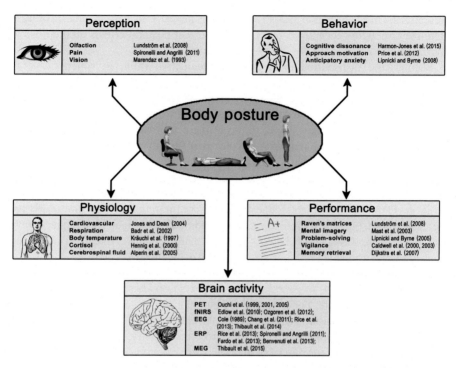

Figure 10.1 Posture modulates physiology and cognition: Select experimental findings. From Thibault, R. T., & Raz, A. (2016). Imaging posture veils neural signals. Frontiers in human neuroscience, 10, 520.

Beyond the psychological and basic physiological measures, posture also exerts a quantifiable and direct impact on brain activity. When we sit upright, our brains assume a different baseline state than when we lie down. Sitting amplifies high-frequency brain waves, associated with alertness and sensory processing, and dampens down low-frequency waves, associated with relaxed or drowsy states [14]. Further studies suggest that posture can influence a core brain system known as the default mode network [15]. Depending on body position, our neurons also respond differently to visual presentations [16], painful stimuli [3], and emotional events [17]. Whereas the majority of these studies employ healthy young adults, posture may exert a particularly strong influence on brain function in the elderly and specific patient groups. Taken together, these insights raise the question: How do we better account for the brain as a component of a body in an environment, thus interpreting neuroimaging results in a fuller context?

By looking at posture in particular, scientists have already made headway on this issue and identified at least three mechanisms by which posture influences brain data. First, lying down may hinder the brain from releasing the chemical precursor to adrenalin. Gravitational loads redistribute when lying down, stimulating receptors in our circulatory system and initiating a physiological cascade that reduces the excitability of neurons. A cleverly designed experiment supports this explanation.

Researchers used inflatable pants to apply leg pressure to participants in order to stabilize circulatory receptor activity and found that postural effects on brain waves were partially negated [9].

Second, the distribution of the highly conductive fluid, in which our brain bathes, differs based on the posture we assume. This substance, known as cerebrospinal fluid, drastically alters electrical signals as they pass from brain to imaging sensor [18]. One study found that when lying face-up, rather than lying face-down, gravity draws the brain downward, thins out the cerebrospinal fluid under posterior brain regions, and in turn, amplifies the electrical signals recorded from the back of the brain [16].

Third, our brains may only be prepared to act on the subset of possible interactions we can have with the surrounding environment based on our current body position. Planning movements depend on the configuration of our limbs [19] and we react more quickly to moving visual fields when upright [20]. Lying down, moreover, decreases social behaviors [21] and hardly invites typical social interactions known to modulate brain activity, such as eye contact [22].

Adopting experimental designs that evaluate and integrate these three mechanisms will refine our ability to use experimental contexts to understand human brain function during everyday life. For example, to help maintain a more "upright" brain state when participants lie down, researchers could entertain the possibility of applying pressure to the body to maintain circulatory receptor activity, pharmacologically sustaining adrenalin levels, or providing periodic stimulation via conversation or sensory input. To overcome variations in the distribution of cerebrospinal fluid, we may require anatomical brain scans from each participant alongside novel compensatory algorithms that cancel out the influence this fluid has on brain signals. Researchers could furthermore weed out participants suffering from sleep-deprivation or other conditions that may cause their brain and body to react differently when upright compared with when lying down. With diligence, neuroimagers can improve current research paradigms to account for a number of these postural discrepancies.

Researchers can also leverage smaller, lighter, and more mobile imaging devices. With the use of overhead tracks, participants undergoing EEG and fNIRS can now move and interact in a laboratory environment. Recent developments, moreover, permit individuals to connect EEG electrodes to their smartphone and record brain activity in everyday contexts [23]. Moving while recording EEG, however, comes with caveats and raises the concern that researchers who are not careful may mistake artifacts for brain oscillations themselves. These portable devices currently sacrifice signal quality for ecological human functioning. Fortunately, technologies can also be used in tandem with one another. In a single experiment, we can combine concurrent data from the more precise and static imaging modalities with data from ecological yet coarser resolution measurements. Similar to how portable devices transformed the field of eye-tracking, wearable neuroimaging technologies may revolutionize how we study the living human brain.

In summary, posture reliably influences brain, body, and mind. This reality rings alarm bells in a field that rarely considers postural constraints. Whereas humans perform the largest diversity of their interactions with the world when standing and moving, most neuroimaging studies demand that participants sit up or lie down and remain motionless. This state of affairs points toward a critical question to ask when interpreting *any* research: How generalizable are the findings? Does the experimental context diverge substantially from an everyday setting? If so, we best interpret the results with due diligence.

Additional readings

A proposal for an embodied approach to neuroscience: Kiverstein J, Miller M. The embodied brain: towards a radical embodied cognitive neuroscience. Front Hum Neurosci 2015;9:1−11.

A landmark research experiment on posture and EEG: Rice JK, Rorden C, Little JS, Parra LC. Subject position affects EEG magnitudes. NeuroImage 2013;64:476−84.

A more in-depth review: Thibault RT, Raz A. Imaging posture veils neural signals. Front Hum Neurosci 2016;10:520.

Section III

The devil's in the details

The replication challenge: Is brain imaging next?

David Mehler

The concept of replication is simple. Do you remember high-school chemistry class —mixing compounds to create explosions? Whether you knew it or not, you were engaged in an attempt to replicate the findings of previous scientists. Unlike these pedagogic experiments, researchers now increasingly attempt to confirm the veracity of findings with carefully crafted and meticulously executed replication studies.

In psychology, for example, a collaboration of unprecedented size set out to replicate 100 highly influential behavioral studies [1]. They successfully replicated 39. As for the remaining 61 studies, we can't be certain whether the original results represent true effects. While these problems of replication have likely existed for decades, only recently have scientists become highly aware of them and realized that—ironically—one of the most replicable findings across the life sciences is the difficulty of replication itself! In the field of brain imaging,

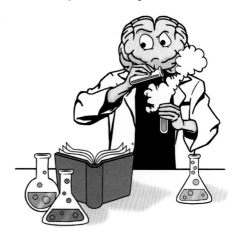

which has considerably fewer replication studies than psychology, researchers have begun to understand why our field may suffer from a similar syndrome. This chapter discusses the forces behind low replicability, including publication bias and researcher bias, and then highlights how adopting an incentive system that encourages high-quality research practices can help overcome these issues.

While some neuroimaging findings seem robust enough to forego formal replication attempts, others could use a second look. For example, motor areas will reliably activate during movement and the amygdala (an area involved in processing fear) will surely respond to fearful stimuli. For several reasons, however, we can't be so certain that more complex analyses such as brain−behavior relationships and contrasts between participants will replicate [2] (e.g., patients compared to healthy

Casting Light on the Dark Side of Brain Imaging. DOI: https://doi.org/10.1016/B978-0-12-816179-1.00010-4

controls). First, head motion, respiration, and heartbeats all contaminate brain recordings and require meticulous removal before analyzing the data [3] and performing statistical analyses [4] (see Chapter 9). Researchers may mistake this noise for a neural signal, especially in "resting state" studies which observe spontaneous brain activity (see Chapter 23). Second, publication bias, researcher bias, and low statistical power all decrease the probability that positive findings represent true effects [5]. *Meta-research*—an entire field in its own right—studies these phenomena and their implications.

Unlike most media reports we hear these days, the press on brain imaging tends to be quite positive. This trend may emerge from *publication bias*—where positive findings are much more likely to reach publication than null results [6]. And yet, null results aren't necessarily the bad news that many people cut them out to be; they may be as informative as positive results. They can tell researchers that the phenomenon they are testing for may not exist after all and that their time can be better spent elsewhere. There are several reasons for publication bias. For instance, researchers may not submit negative findings for publication because the results contradict their prior beliefs and journals tend to decline the publication of null findings more often than positive results [7]—both examples of what scientists call the *file drawer effect*. Thus the published literature may merely represent the "tip of the iceberg" [8]. A massive amount of research may never surface, and in turn, never inform future experiments. How we report scientific findings appears to matter more than previously thought.

Another factor, *researcher bias*, also reduces replicability. This term encompasses various questionable research practices, including selectively presenting results that fit a preferred storyline and omitting information that would allow others to replicate an experiment. Investigators often adopt questionable research practices unintentionally, but at times they may also intentionally modify their analyses to push statistical results beyond the widely accepted line that scientists use to define findings as significant (so called *p-hacking*) [9]. One common example is when researchers perform many statistical tests on one dataset but fail to account for the fact that running more tests means that there will be a higher chance of obtaining spurious results. Every test is associated with a probability for a false positive, also called the *error rate*. In other words, test results may suggest that there is an effect although in reality no effect exists—that we are chasing ghosts. Statistical error rates increase with the number of tests conducted, so adjusting for multiple tests becomes especially important in brain imaging experiments, where researchers often perform thousands of tests on one dataset. Neuroimagers are still working out how to best adjust for multiple tests within complex analyses [4].

Clear reporting of methods is particularly important in brain imaging research. Take a guess at how many ways we can analyze data from a single brain scan. Theoretically countless, practically at least 69,000 different ways! [10]. Functional brain images aren't photographs. They are statistical maps resulting from complex digital image manipulation and analyses. In fact, brain imaging data usually require between 6 and 10 steps of general data preparation and analysis. Researchers can perform each of these steps in a variety of ways, regardless of whether the data comes from functional magnetic resonance imaging (fMRI), electroencephalogram, magnetoencephalogram, or other imaging techniques. Different choices in data processing and analysis can lead to widely divergent results: small variations can quickly sum to form large discrepancies [10,11]. In some cases, researchers may run many variations of an analysis, but only report results that support their hypotheses. This practice can lead to biased publications that overestimate true effects [12]. The third major cause of poor replicability—low statistical power—is addressed in detail in the following chapter.

Now that we have covered the forces driving the publication of false positives, let's focus on how to remedy the problem. Current reward structures in academia—including job promotions and funding schemes—primarily incentivize publishing articles in esteemed academic journals. These high impact journals are much more interested in novel and glossy findings compared to replication efforts. Hence, the reward structure and publication system partly reinforce the status quo: scientists are incentivized to focus on positive findings and work with underpowered studies that consume fewer resources [13]. Further, they are encouraged to investigate novel effects, rather than retest old findings. In fact, such incentives may be one reason why scientists rarely design costly neuroimaging experiments with replication in mind. Overall, current reward structures largely fail to promote high-quality science.

What can neuroscientists learn from the replication challenge to make their work more replicable? Beyond more rigorous training in experimental design and statistics, one growing research practice may be game-changing—and that is the preregistration of the methods, analyses, and aims of an experiment before data collection even begins. This documentation is often stored on an openly accessible platform such as *clinicaltrials.gov* or the open science framework (OSF). Another option is to submit a *registered-report* where peer-reviewers assess the rationale for the study design, its proposed methods, and the planned statistical power before data are collected [14]. As long as authors follow their protocol, accepted registered reports are guaranteed to be published irrespective of the final results. Researchers can also upload open access versions of their articles before they reach publication, known as preprints. This procedure can allow for informal and transparent feedback, and hence an open discussion of the research. Altogether, preregistration, registered reports, and preprints help address the three main issues underlying the replication challenge: publication bias, researcher bias, and low statistical power.

In addition to collecting new data to *replicate* findings, scientists should also be able to reperform reported analysis on an existing dataset to *reproduce* results [11]. While replication studies are still relatively rare in neuroimaging (partly because imaging experiments are costly, but also because there are more incentives to study new research questions than probe previous ones), journals have recently published a number of insightful reproduction studies that used openly available data sets. Various factors influence how well results can be reproduced. These include the quality of documentation, potential errors in the original analyses, the robustness of the statistical effect [15], and even the software package used [16]. The more steps analyses comprise, the more likely errors can occur and sum up. Notably, the

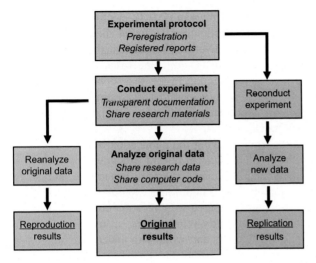

Figure 11.1 Depicts an original experiment (gold), a reproduction attempt (gray), and a replication attempt (orange). Whereas reproductions re-analyze the original data, replications re-conduct the original experimental protocol and analyze new data. Steps that can be taken to increase subsequent reproduction and replication success are listed in italics.

prestige of a journal falls short as a guarantor for the reliability of its findings. On the contrary, journal prestige may be associated with below-average reproducibility [17]. Only transparent reporting of methods, analyses, code, and data makes research more reproducible and hence represents best scientific practice [18].

Fortunately, the field of neuroimaging is witnessing rapid and promising efforts to improve the quality and robustness of its findings. Like research in psychology and genetics, neuroimagers are setting new standards with several open data projects (e.g., the human connectome project, open fMRI, and the Enhancing Neuro Imaging Genetics through Meta-Analysis (ENIGMA) consortium) [11]. Neuroscientists can use these open data sets to test parameters, validate analyses, and address new research questions [2,4,11]. They can also use these data to estimate the number of participants needed to render neuroimaging results replicable [19]. Altogether, these initiatives leave room for optimism. As the field moves toward more rigorous methodology, we can benefit from noting that replicating experiments alone can only tell us so much [20]. Instead, multiple lines of evidence from experiments that deliberately use different methods while addressing the same research question, known as *hypothesis generalizability*, are likely even more fruitful to advance science.

In summary, the replication challenge urges scientists across disciplines to overcome biases and maximize freely available access to their work in order to encourage independent researchers to test and verify published results. In doing so, researchers can benefit from openly sharing their hypotheses and experimental methods from the start. The field of neuroimaging in particular has started to address the replication challenge by developing best practice guidelines, software for reproducible science, and databases for preregistration and open science [11]. These developments will likely transform the way we image brains, and when combined with new technology, lead to promising breakthroughs.

Acknowledgments

The author acknowledges Dr. Chris Allen, Dr. Chris Chambers, Dr. Russell Poldrack, and Johannes Algermissen for insightful discussions on the topic, which have inspired parts of this chapter.

Additional readings

An in-depth review of questionable research practices and solutions to the replication crisis: Chambers C. The seven deadly sins of psychology: a manifesto for reforming the culture of scientific practice. Princeton university Press; 2017.

A landmark replication study in psychology, the Open Science Project: Collaboration OS. Estimating the reproducibility of psychological science. Science (80-) 2015;349(6251): aac4716.

A comprehensive review on reproducible neuroimaging: Poldrack RA, Baker CI, Durnez J, et al. Scanning the horizon: towards transparent and reproducible neuroimaging research. Nat Rev Neurosci 2017;18(2):115−26.

Power and design considerations in imaging research

12

Marcus R. Munafò, Henk R. Cremers, Tor D. Wager and Tal Yarkoni

Why should we care about statistical power? It turns out that many research findings may be false, and low power is one of the main culprits [1]. Low power, by definition, reduces the probability of discovering real effects. In other words, compared to well-powered studies, underpowered studies produce more false negatives—they conclude no effect exists when in reality one does. However, low statistical power also undermines the reliability of research findings in two less-appreciated ways. First, it reduces the probability that an observation passing the threshold for claiming discovery (i.e., statistical significance) actually reflects a real effect. Second, it can lead to an exaggerated estimate of the magnitude of an effect. This effect inflation is sometimes referred to as the "Winner's Curse," the analogy being an auction, where the winner typically pays an inflated price. It often occurs when researchers claim a discovery based on thresholds (e.g., statistical significance, or a Bayes factor of a given value; see additional readings for a more detailed

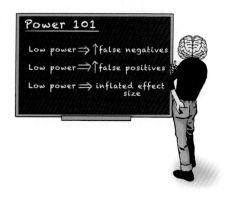

description of these issues) [2,3]. In this chapter, we highlight not only the causes and consequences of low statistical power, but also how functional magnetic resonance imaging (fMRI) researchers are addressing these issues and why we can remain hopeful.

The concept of statistical power is intrinsically linked to the Null Hypothesis Significance Testing (NHST) framework that continues to dominate the biomedical sciences. We can, however, frame the problem in other ways. For instance, some researchers encourage a taxonomy that discusses errors of inference in terms of magnitude (Type M) and sign (Type S) [4], rather than the standard false positive (Type 1) and false negative (Type 2) used in the NHST framework. Smaller sample sizes, all other things being equal, will increase the risk of errors for

Casting Light on the Dark Side of Brain Imaging. DOI: https://doi.org/10.1016/B978-0-12-816179-1.00011-6

both magnitude and sign—in other words, estimates are more likely to deviate substantially from the true population effect, and also more likely to be in the opposite direction [4]. This is linked to the concept of "vibration of effects" [2]— the tendency of small, underpowered studies to be imprecise and therefore provide a wide range of estimates around the true effect size. This is particularly problematic when stringent significance thresholds and publication bias against "null" results conspire to select only the extremes of that range for publication.

Researchers have attempted to estimate the average statistical power of studies across the biomedical sciences. This endeavor remains challenging due to the difficulty in estimating the magnitude of "true" effects (because what is published is only a proportion of all the work conducted, and because of factors such as the Winner's Curse which means these published estimates will be imprecise and potentially inflated). Conventionally, scientists aim for at least 80% power (i.e., a 20% chance of accepting a false negative). Evidence suggests, however, that average power is considerably lower. Within the neurosciences, researchers revealed that average power ranges between $\sim 8\%$ and $\sim 31\%$ [2]—although the distribution may depend on the study type and methodology [5]. These numbers mean that somewhere between 69% and 92% of true effects go undetected. This pattern replicates across a wider range of biomedical sciences [6]. In the neuroimaging literature, estimating effect sizes is even more complex. Nonetheless, a summary of 1131 fMRI studies conducted over a span of more than 20 years suggests that sample sizes have increased only modestly in this time. As of 2015, the median fMRI study was only powered to detect large effect sizes ($d = 0.75$; [7,8]), whereas the typical effect size for the phenomena being tested is likely to be smaller ($d = 0.50$; [7]). Moreover, these estimates come from studies with relatively high-power compared to most fMRI studies [9]. In other words, most fMRI studies don't include enough participants to detect the effects they seek using the standard NHST approach.

Causes and consequence of low power in functional magnetic resonance imaging research

Low statistical power is a problem for any type of research, but certain aspects of fMRI research make the power problem more prominent, and the consequences more troublesome. Here, we elucidate at least three prominent causes with a simple example. Imagine we are conducting an fMRI study on working memory and want to compare patients with a major depressive disorder (MDD) to a group of healthy controls. First, the standard way of analyzing fMRI data divides the brain into about a hundred thousand small cubes, termed "voxels," and looks at the data from each voxel independently. This so-called *mass univariate* analysis requires adjusting the significance threshold (for instance from $P < .05$ to $P < .0001$) in order to keep the probability of a false positive low, but this stringent threshold requirement necessarily reduces statistical power. Second, the sample size in fMRI studies has only risen modestly over the years [7] despite increasing awareness of the power problem for both functional and structural MRI [2]. In contrast to genetic research, where costs have fallen dramatically enough to allow for high-powered studies, fMRI research remains fairly expensive (around $500 per hour of scanner use) and these fees are unlikely to drop substantially anytime soon. This price tag limits the acquisition of large samples, and in addition, clinical samples, like MDD patients, are difficult to recruit. These first two causes of low statistical power—adjusted statistical thresholds and cost—would not be a major concern if the (expected) effect sizes were very large. However, it is becoming increasingly clear that effect sizes in fMRI are in the low to medium range, and this issue represents the third cause of low statistical power in fMRI research. Some of the large effect sizes in the fMRI literature may emerge due to selective publication of positive results (publication bias, [8]) and the selection of participants who are not representative of the wider population (sampling bias, [9]), or a combination of both. Of course, effect size varies by domain, research question, design, and other factors; however, researchers are realizing that extremely large effects in fMRI research—which would be required to achieve conventional statistical significance with current sample sizes—are rare. Novel approaches (described in the following section) may substantially increase power by increasing effect sizes.

As mentioned in the introduction, the consequences of low statistical power extend beyond its definition—a high chance of missing true effects. Some researchers may consider the increase in the false negative rate as an acceptable trade-off to control the false positive rate. However, the three causes of low power which we describe earlier (large number of dependent variables, small sample sizes, and small effect sizes) have at least three less-appreciated, but potentially far-reaching, consequences. First, as noted earlier, the combination of a small sample size and stringent significance threshold induces a large potential for inflation of statistically significant effects. Therefore effect sizes reported in fMRI studies with relatively small samples can be highly inflated, or even in the opposite direction of, the true effect [3]. In our example, we might find a difference in prefrontal activity between the MDD and control group. When we plot the extracted data of that region, the difference may look spectacularly large. However, this is most likely a case of the described winner's curse and the true effects are much smaller. Second, this potential effect size inflation, in combination with the availability of many dependent variables, can easily lead to misleading inferences about the neural architecture of cognition [9]. In particular, when true effects are small and diffusely distributed throughout the brain (a plausible model for many cognitive processes and differences between psychiatric patients and control groups), underpowered studies will tend to identify only a small subset of effects, but with substantially inflated effect sizes—often leading researchers to incorrectly conclude that effects are strong and localized. When looking at the statistical map comparing the MDD patients and control group, we may observe just one or perhaps a few "spots" in the brain—yet the true difference in neural functioning between the two groups is much more likely to be distributed and small. Third, a consequence of low power is that different studies on the same psychological process and/or psychiatric disorder will report disparate results. One study might report a strong difference between MDD and controls in one region, another study an effect in a completely different region, so that the second doesn't replicate the first. This situation requires no explanation other than low power (although low power is rarely the first explanation a researcher will reach for) [2], and it is exacerbated by various forms of reporting bias [8], making it extremely difficult to achieve robust cross-study consensus.

Potential solutions and future directions

Fortunately, there are several solutions to the power problem in fMRI research. The most straightforward way to increase statistical power is to increase the sample size. This practice, of course, is easier said than done: fMRI scanning is expensive, and the recruitment of specific populations difficult (e.g., psychiatric patients). If we strive to maintain the conventional standard of a 5% chance of having at least one false positive among many analyses (termed full family-wise error rate correction), we would need hundreds of participants—particularly for between-groups comparisons (such as our MDD example) and analyses of individual differences [10]. Some scientists are tackling this problem head-on and initiating large-multicenter collaborations and building publicly available fMRI databases [7].

Another straightforward but controversial means to increase statistical power is to apply a more lenient statistical significance threshold. The argument here is that if true effects are small and distributed across the brain, we would need a lenient significance threshold to detect them. The controversy surrounding this approach stems from the parallel increase in false positives. This practice becomes hard to justify when chosing a threshold that increases statistical power just enough to detect at least one statistically significant effect [9].

A third way to increase statistical power is to apply a "region of interest" (ROI) approach, where researchers focus on a single brain region, chosen a priori, instead of all brain regions. Using an ROI approach, we can avoid the need to statistically correct for thousands of voxels, and in turn increase the statistical power. However, there is a great deal of flexibility in how one defines a region [10], and substantial uncertainty in whether a certain region was truly chosen a priori. This potential for "hypothesizing after results are known," or HARKing [7], limits the conclusions that we can draw. Preregistrating study protocols, and prespecifying regions of interest, can help address this limitation (see previous chapter for more details).

Finally, testing each voxel often yields low power and focusing only on ROIs might miss other relevant areas of the brain. An emerging family of measures test predefined patterns that involve multiple variables distributed across many brain regions and/or systems to address both these concern. For example, rather than testing 20 or so regions involved in working memory, you can define one a priori pattern across the images and test the "expression of" or response in that pattern. In the simplest terms, this would involve taking the average activity in the regions included in the pattern. One recent study, for example, did just this [11]. The researchers used neurosynth [12] to identify a working memory-related pattern, averaged over this pattern to develop a single measure of working memory-related activity, and then tested that single measure for effects of a psychosocial stressor [11]. Another recent study has extended this concept to test averages over predefined large-scale networks [13]. This example looked at seven predefined cortical networks [14] that span the cortex. This approach largely reduces bias and the potential for HARKing. Moreover, limiting the analysis to seven patterns reduces the problem of multiple comparisons.

Multivariate pattern-based approaches can also yield much greater effect sizes, and reduce the number of tests from many voxels to the expression of a single, predefined pattern [15,16]. For example, when researchers applied an established multivariate pattern—a pain-predictive model called the Neurologic Pain Signature [17] —to new individual participants, they found very large effect sizes for high versus low pain ($d = 1.2-3.50$) [17,18]. Similarly, a negative emotion-predictive model, the Picture Induced Negative Emotion Signature [19], differentiated emotionally negative images from neutral images with an effect size of $d = 4.69$. Effect sizes for a Vicarious Pain Signature [18], applied to comparisons of high versus low observed pain in independent samples, ranged from $d = 1.63-1.75$ [18,20]. These effect sizes are several times larger than those found in voxel-wise analyses [7], and do not require correction for multiple comparisons when testing the magnitude of the response in a pattern as a whole. These examples illustrate that novel analytic approaches can address statistical power concerns and provide biomarkers for cognitive and affective processes that can be validated and used across studies.

Conclusions

More and more researchers are beginning to appreciate the implications of low statistical power, from the need for a priori sample size calculations to inform study design, to the impact of low power on the robustness of a study's conclusions. In the context of fMRI, high costs, small effect sizes, small sample sizes, and multiple comparisons all exacerbate the problem of low statistical power. Fortunately, brain researchers are increasingly addressing the issue of low power using both solutions that apply to the wider scientific enterprise, as well as a number of fMRI-specific advances, including novel analytical approaches. Taken together, we can remain cautiously optimistic that the robustness of the fMRI literature will improve.

Additional readings

Button KS, Ioannidis JP, Mokrysz C, Nosek BA, Flint J, Robinson ES, et al. Power failure: why small sample size undermines the reliability of neuroscience. Nat Rev Neurosci 2013;14(5):365−76. PubMed PMID: 23571845.

Poldrack RA, Baker CI, Durnez J, Gorgolewski KJ, Matthews PM, Munafo MR, et al. Scanning the horizon: towards transparent and reproducible neuroimaging research. Nat Rev Neurosci 2017;18(2):115−26. PubMed PMID: 28053326.

Why neuroimaging can't diagnose autism

13

Robert T. Thibault, Lauren Dahl and Amir Raz

Wouldn't it be convenient if you could scan your toddler's brain to test for autism? Or, if you're feeling stressed out and down, to neuroimage your own head and see if you're just going through a phase or whether you have clinical anxiety or depression? What about scanning for schizophrenia, bipolar disorder, obsessive compulsive disorder, or any other mental condition for that matter? If we had this ability, the implications would be widespread and the benefits tangible.

Unfortunately, this option just isn't available yet. Some media reports, however, suggest that the day of diagnostic neuroimaging may be right around the corner. These promises often stem from studies where researchers successfully distinguish between individuals with and without mental conditions: for example, identifying brain scans from people with conditions such as autism spectrum disorder (ASD), major depressive disorder, and schizophrenia with 80%−90% accuracy [1].

With this level of precision, is it only a matter of time before widespread adoption of diagnostic neuroimaging? Not so fast. A simple, but often overlooked, nuance stands in our way. And that nuance lies in the word *accuracy*. Accuracy has both a vague usage in common speech and a very specific meaning in medical diagnoses. Let's use a real life example to illustrate the importance of the different uses of this term [2].

Not too long ago, the physicist Leonard Mlodinow (who notably wrote *A Briefer History of Time* with Stephen Hawking) applied for life insurance and had his blood drawn. As life insurance companies do, they wanted to ensure Mlodinow didn't have any life-threatening illness before insuring him. Surprisingly, the company denied his application for life insurance. Mlodinow's doctor confirmed that he tested positive for HIV and that the test was 99.9% accurate. And yet, Mlodinow remained calm, knowing that this "accuracy" meant he had only a 9% chance of truly being HIV positive.

Wait a second... The doctor says the test is 99.9% accurate and Mlodinow interprets this as a 9% chance of having HIV. What's going on? Fortunately, we don't

Casting Light on the Dark Side of Brain Imaging. DOI: https://doi.org/10.1016/B978-0-12-816179-1.00012-8

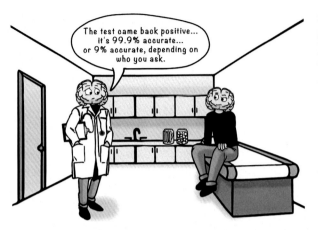

The test came back positive... it's 99.9% accurate... or 9% accurate, depending on who you ask.

need to be brilliant theoretical physicists of the Mlodinow caliber to understand why he didn't flinch at the test results. The discrepancy between the 99.9% and the 9% manifests because few people in his demographic actually have HIV—the prevalence, or "base rate" is low, about 1 in 10,000, or 0.01%. To use technical terms, the HIV test has a "specificity" of 99.9% (the likelihood that the test appears negative given that the person doesn't have HIV) and a "positive predictive value" of about 9% (the likelihood that the person has HIV given that the test is positive). To better understand this issue, let's look at Table 13.1. It illustrates the outcome of HIV tests on 1,000,000 people of Mlodinow's demographic. While we've included a complete table for those who want a deeper understanding of the issue, we highlighted in yellow the important terms such as base rate, specificity, positive predictive value, and their associated percentages.

As you can see, results from this type of medical test require a bit of interpretation. Both Mlodinow and his doctor were correct; they were simply reporting different statistics: Mlodinow focused on the positive predictive value; his doctor on specificity. In this scenario the positive predictive value constitutes the much more interesting percentage. Once Mlodinow receives a positive test result, he knows the

Table 13.1 Diagnostic chart for a population of 1,000,000 who were HIV tested

Total (1,000,000)	People with HIV (100)	People without HIV (999,900)	Base rate $\frac{100}{1,000,000} = 0.01\%$
Tested positive (1,095)	True positive (95)	False positive (1000)	Positive predictive value $\frac{95}{1095} = 9\%$
Tested negative (998,905)	False negative (5)	True negative (998,900)	Negative predictive value $\frac{998,900}{998,905} > 99.99\%$
	Sensitivity $\frac{95}{100} = 95\%$	Specificity $\frac{998,900}{999,900} = 99.9\%$	

These tests are commonly considered 99.9% accurate (specificity); meanwhile, the 9% positive predictive value represents a more interesting statistic for those who test positive.

result can only be a true positive or a false positive. Looking at specificity tells him little; looking at the positive predictive value tells him how likely it is that he actually has HIV.[1]

This example almost touches on the true technical diagnostic definition of accuracy: the total number of correctly classified cases divided by the total number of cases (in our example, $95 + 998,900$ divided by $1,000,000$). For conditions with low base rates the percentage associated with accuracy is often very close to that indicated by specificity. In our example, accuracy is a hair less than 99.9%. In different contexts the word "accuracy" could loosely indicate specificity, the positive predictive value, sensitivity (the likelihood that a test is positive given that the person has the condition) or, the correct technical definition. Now that we've hashed out the statistical concept, let's turn back to diagnostic brain imaging.

By looking at brain scans, researchers can distinguish between individuals with and without ASD with up to 90% accuracy. But does this mean I can bring my toddler to a brain imaging clinic and find out whether she has ASD? As for the HIV example, we need to first determine the base rate for ASD (which is somewhere between 1% and 2%) [3,4]. Now we can flesh out the same Table 13.1 and work backward to calculate the value we are interested in—the positive predictive value. We'll use the results from a widely reported diagnostic neuroimaging study on ASD [5], which has previously been dissected in the *Guardian* [6], for our Table 13.2.

The positive predictive value is about 4%. That means, if we use this test (which legitimately has greater than 80% accuracy in technical terms) for every child correctly diagnosed with ASD, another 24 will be incorrectly diagnosed with ASD. To have a very good positive predictive value, we would need to either look at a condition with a much higher base rate or have very high accuracy (or both). However, given the behavioral and neurological heterogeneity of most psychiatric conditions (outlined in Chapter 3), nearing 100% accuracy may present an intractable task.

As you will appreciate next, whether or not we should use diagnostic neuroimaging depends on much more than the positive predictive value alone. Imagine a scenario where an initial brain scan could identify the development of a tumor with a positive predictive value of 4%. If the 96 out of the 100 people who are incorrectly diagnosed with a brain tumor could immediately go through another test to confirm whether the initial scan was a true positive, little harm would be done. If the remaining four people correctly diagnosed could now receive a treatment to remove the tumor before it causes any serious issues, large benefits would ensue. In this scenario a positive predictive value of 4% could be sufficient to recommend the test. In the case of ASD, individuals incorrectly diagnosed with ASD (or rather their parents) may suffer considerable stress until the child is old enough to test for ASD behaviorally. There's no clear route of further action to take for those correctly diagnosed. Thus in the case of ASD the harms of using a test with a low positive predictive value seem to outweigh the benefits.

---

[1] In case you're wondering, further tests confirmed that Mlodinow did not have HIV.

Table 13.2 Key diagnostic values for neuroimaging ASD

Total (1000)	People with ASD (10)	People without ASD (990)	Base rate $\frac{10}{1000} = 1\%$
Tested positive (207)	True positive (9)	False positive (198)	Positive predictive value $\frac{9}{207} = 4\%$
Tested negative (793)	False negative (1)	True negative (792)	Negative predictive value $\frac{792}{793} = 99.9\%$
	Sensitivity $\frac{9}{10} = 90\%$	Specificity $\frac{792}{990} = 80\%$	

While researchers and clinicians continue to conduct studies to improve diagnostic neuroimaging toward a clinically useful state, some practitioners claim that they can already provide this service (see Chapter 22). These declarations have been rejected by major clinical societies and research experts, but these rebukes haven't stopped such practitioners from becoming wealthy at the expense of gullible clients. While diagnostic neuroimaging for psychiatric conditions may well find a place in the future of medicine, it likely won't look anything like today's private clinics. Unfortunately, for these private practitioners, terms such as sensitivity, specificity, and positive predictive value are of little concern.

When discussing the results of any diagnostic test, it can be helpful to think not only of the percentages, but more importantly, precisely what those percentages mean. It could just save you some distress at your next visit to the doctor.

Additional readings

A breezy academic article on diagnostic probabilities: Gigerenzer G, Edwards A. Simple tools for understanding risks: from innumeracy to insight. BMJ 2003;327(7417):741–4.

A well written and popular style book on randomness and statistics: Mlodinow L. The drunkard's walk: how randomness rules our lives. Vintage; 2009.

Section IV

Neuroimaging: Holy Grail or false prophet?

From mind to brain: The challenge of neuro-reductionism

14

Ian Gold

Science is a mosaic. Theories are developed to answer particular questions—*What are the building blocks of the universe? How do organisms reproduce? What causes earthquakes?* These questions tend to be concerned with particular objects and processes at various scales—subatomic particles, such as quarks and their combinations, DNA and replication, the earth's crust and its movement. Typically, there are gaps in the conceptual spaces between theories. Although we may have a fairly good idea of how quarks combine to form hadrons and how nucleotides are conjoined into DNA molecules, no theory is currently concerned with relating hadrons to DNA, though of course we believe that some story of composition could be told in principle.

Sometimes, however, scientific theories manage to bridge the conceptual gaps. The field of molecular genetics provides a paradigmatic example. Until the discovery of the structure of the DNA molecule, no theory provided an account of reproduction in molecular terms. Once geneticists realized that what the older genetic theory of Mendel referred to as the "gene" was in fact (roughly) a DNA molecule, they were able to span the gap between molecules and genes and provide an account of inheritance in molecular terms. This discovery resulted in the "reduction" of Mendelian theory to molecular genetics.

According to the classical account (associated with the philosopher Ernest Nagel [1]), reduction occurs when one scientific theory—the "reducing" theory—is capable of deriving the laws of another scientific theory—the "reduced" theory—along with some definitions linking the theories. So, for example, once it was possible to construct definitions of the form "'gene' is identical to 'DNA molecule,'" molecular genetic theory had the conceptual resources to generate the laws of Mendelian genetics and thereby reduce it.

Reductionism has played a prominent role in discussions about the relations among the sciences of the mind. When we speak of reductionism in this context, we typically mean the view that psychological theories (and perhaps theories of human behavior found in anthropology, sociology, economics, and the like) will be reduced to neuroscientific theories. By analogy with the case of genetics mentioned earlier, when a neuroscientific (reducing) theory is capable of generating the laws of a psychological (reduced) theory, we could declare the reduction of psychology to neuroscience accomplished. This would require similarly linking definitions like

Casting Light on the Dark Side of Brain Imaging. DOI: https://doi.org/10.1016/B978-0-12-816179-1.00013-X

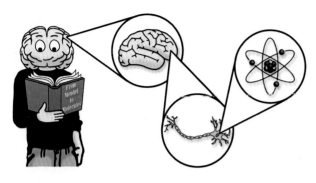

"'learning' (of such-and-such a type) is identical to synaptic plasticity (of such-and-such a type)." Whether the psychological sciences would retain any role remains unclear. The philosophers Paul M. Churchland and Patricia S. Churchland [2,3] have argued that the psychological sciences are so conceptually flawed that a successful neuroscientific account of the mind would motivate an elimination of psychology altogether.

Although neuroscience is still a very young science, large portions of the scientific community, and even the general public, believe that neuroscientific theory will eventually reduce psychological theory. How plausible is this view? In order to answer that question, we have to know why so many people believe in neural reduction in the first place. Surprisingly, an explicit defense of this view is hard to come by. One of the likelier explanations is that many people assume reduction is inevitable, simply because they accept that the mind is nothing more than the functioning brain. Accordingly, it would seem obvious that successful theories of the mind *must be* theories of the brain. What else could they be? Unfortunately, we cannot predict the future course of science with nearly the degree of confidence that this simple argument might lead us to believe. Even if the mind were nothing over and above the brain, this fact would no more guarantee that successful theories of the mind will be theories of the brain than the fact that DNA molecules are constituted of hadrons guarantees that a final theory of reproduction will come from fundamental physics. Although genes are undoubtedly constituted of hadrons, scientists may remain unable to produce a hadron theory of genes. Even if such a theory *could* be produced, it stands a good chance of being less elegant, useful, or illuminating than the molecular theory. Brains, like genes, are made up of hadrons, or whatever particles physics eventually identifies as basic. And yet few if any scientists foresee a successful theory of color vision, or long-term memory, or mind-wandering that will make reference to hadrons, though such a theory is certainly within the realm of possibilities. Only the actual course of science will determine whether psychology reduces to neuroscience. At present, we have no good reason to anticipate the imminent arrival of such a development.

An analogous confusion arises *within* neuroscience when one thinks about the particular kind of neuroscientific theory that is likely to illuminate the features of mental life. Not long ago the distinguished neuroscientist Horace Barlow [4] proposed that single neurons were the optimal level at which to understand psychological phenomena (at least perceptual phenomena). That is no longer the case. Neuroscientists now widely believe that cognition is likely to depend on neural circuitry in relatively large or diffuse regions of the brain. As a result, brain imaging, rather than single cell neurophysiology, is now the favored neuroscientific methodology for understanding mental function. There is certainly reason to think that both single neurons and neural circuitry will contribute to our understanding of cognition. But what would lead us to think that the current assumption that circuitry is the right level is any better justified now than the single unit doctrine was in the 1970s? Indeed, we might wonder whether it isn't in fact the *availability* of the technology that makes circuits seem so illuminating now as single cells seemed then. Just as it is premature to believe that science *must* evolve toward a reduction of psychology to neuroscience, it is premature to assume that the contribution of neuroscience to our understanding of the mind must be at one level of neural organization rather than some other.

A belief in reduction, then, is something of an ideology in the sciences of the mind rather than a description of actual scientific progress. Indeed, reduction is rare in any branch of science, even in physics where, as the philosopher Tim Maudlin [5] has argued, we might expect scientists to find reduction easiest to achieve. And there is no good reason to think that scientists will find reduction easier to achieve in the sciences of the mind, however welcome that achievement might be. While the science of the brain will undoubtedly contribute something to a future theory of the mind, the nature of the theoretical links between descriptions of the brain and descriptions of mental phenomena remains to be discovered.

Further reading

A detailed defense of the reduction of psychology to neuroscience: Bickle J. Psychoneural reduction: the new wave. Cambridge: MIT Press; 1998.

Among the most influential arguments against reductionism: Fodor J. Special sciences: or the disunity of science as a working hypothesis. Synthese 1974;28(2):97−115.

A presentation and critique of some important arguments in support of reductionism: Gold I, Gold I, Stoljar D. A neuron doctrine in the philosophy of neuroscience. Behav Brain Sci 1999;22(5):809−30.

A useful overview of the notion of reduction in science: Van Riel R, Van Gulick R. Scientific reduction. In: Stanford encyclopedia of philosophy; 2014. <https://plato.stanford.edu/entries/scientific-reduction>.

The power of belief in the magic of neuroscience

Jay A. Olson

> *Any sufficiently advanced technology is indistinguishable from magic.*
>
> Arthur C. Clark

Pick a number from 1 to 100. Now imagine that a neuroimaging machine could guess which number you chose or even insert a new number into your head. Would you consider this mind reading and thought insertion to be sufficiently advanced technology—or magic? In this chapter, we'll explore how the allure of neuroscience can hijack our capacity for critical thinking, among lay people and neuroscientists alike.

Over the past few decades, researchers have attempted to uncover the link between neural activation and thoughts. They've made progress in decoding mental content—"mind reading"—using neuroimaging. In one study, for example, participants saw photographs of objects then later imagined them. The researchers could infer which objects the participants were thinking of based on their brain activity alone [1]. These types of procedures, however, are generally slow and error-prone. They work better for distinct and vivid content, such as imagining an owl versus an umbrella, than they do for abstract content such as numbers. Perhaps in another few decades, computers and neuroimaging will be able to instantly determine which number you chose—but we're not there yet.

Progress has been even slower on thought insertion: implanting mental content using brain stimulation. Half a century ago, neurosurgeon Wilder Penfield famously inserted electrodes into patients' brains and caused them to hallucinate and recall various memories. This method, though, is crude and of course invasive. There is presently no way to insert a specific thought, like a number, into one's brain.

But what if we could convince people otherwise? As demonstrated in earlier chapters, people trust neuroscience. Tossing a picture of a brain scan into an article increases its credibility, whether or not it adds anything to the argument [2]. But do people trust neuroscience enough to believe that machines can read their mind or plant thoughts in their head? These were the questions my colleagues and I asked at McGill University [3]. To answer them, we needed a little bit of magic.

In our study, we put 60 undergraduate students in a brain scanner that we said used a new type of neuroimaging technology. After proper calibration the machine could ostensibly read and influence thoughts. To test this, we had participants pick an arbitrary number while inside the scanner. We told them that by reading and

Casting Light on the Dark Side of Brain Imaging. DOI: https://doi.org/10.1016/B978-0-12-816179-1.00015-3

influencing their neural activation patterns, the machine could infer which
number they chose or insert a new
number into their head.

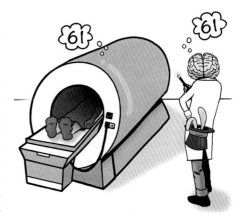

Imagine that you're a participant in
this study. You enter the scanner, and
the experimenter tells you to concentrate
on the number 0, then the number 1, and
so on, all the way up to 9. You lie
motionless in the scanner with your eyes
closed, believing that the machine is calibrating and recording what your brain
looks like while thinking of different
numbers.

You silently choose a number from 1 to 100 then exit the scanner. A printer in
the adjacent control room outputs some complicated statistics and its guess of your
chosen number.

The experimenter brings this sheet into the room and asks you which number
you chose. To your amazement, the numbers match: the machine guessed your
number before you even said it. Somehow, the machine seemed to read your mind.

This was what our participants experienced, but the real magic happened behind
the scenes. The machine was actually a sham: although it resembled a regular scanner, it was actually made of wood and had no functioning parts. Researchers use
these kinds of scanners to get children comfortable before entering real brain scanners, which are larger and more intimidating. A speaker inside the scanner played
MRI noises, like buzzes and beeps, that we had downloaded online.

The printer, too, was a sham: it wasn't even plugged in, nor was any of the
technical-looking equipment. And the machine didn't guess the number. That was
actually a magic trick; the experimenter, played by myself, is a magician. You may
have seen this trick performed on stage in which the magician appears to read an
audience member's mind. Same trick, different context.

After a few trials of this mystical feat, we told participants that we would now
do the reverse: the *machine* would pick a number and influence them to choose it.
How? The machine would activate the areas in the brain associated with that number, as recorded during the calibration phase. If the machine chose the number 42,
it would activate the areas of the participant's brain which were active when thinking of the numbers 4 and 2. The activation occurs using "natural electromagnetic
fluctuations," which are completely safe, we assured participants. If they asked any
questions about these fluctuations, we gave them increasingly convoluted answers
until they stopped asking.

This time, the machine would appear to randomly choose and print out a number, then the experimenter would bring this piece of paper—face down—back into
the brain scanner room. The participant would slide into the machine, choose a
number, then slide out. The experimenter would then flip over the paper to reveal
the participant's number. Again: same trick, different context.

In the first condition, the machine appeared to read the participant's thoughts; in the second, it appeared to influence them. If people trusted this procedure and neuroscience enough, we expected them to believe—and maybe even *feel*—that the machine was doing something to their mind. And that's exactly what we found.

Participants reported less control over their decisions when they believed the machine was influencing them. In fact, they had a plethora of unusual experiences. Several reported that once a number popped into their head, they *could not change* that number. One reported that her eyes darted back and forth without her control while choosing a number, then they stopped when she had selected one. Another claimed that the numbers in his head were not his own; he ended up choosing 61, a number that he particularly disliked and would have never chosen himself. While under the scanner's "influence," one participant reported a throbbing headache, which suddenly disappeared after we debriefed her. At the extreme, one participant even claimed:

> *I feel like it's a voice . . . dragging me from the number that already exists in my mind. I . . . feel some kind of force, or some kind of . . . image, or [something] trying to distract me from this number, and then I form [another one].*

Seeing these results, you may be thinking: "Not me! *I* would never fall for that!" Beware of the cognitive bias called the curse of knowledge, in which once you know something, it seems completely obvious. Our studies have worked on psychology and neuroscience students—including those *explicitly taught* that such technology is currently impossible [4]. It has worked on graduate students in neuroscience, postdoctoral fellows, and neuroimaging researchers. And, had you not read this book, it may have even worked on you.

These studies are not about deception. They're not about fooling people, nor are they about magic. They're about belief. People trust neuroscience enough to let go of their critical thinking and accept that a neuroimaging machine is doing the impossible.

And if this belief is strong enough to remove people's feelings of control over their thoughts, perhaps we can also use it to increase control. If it can give headaches, perhaps it can also remove them. As we'll see next, we can leverage this power of belief in the magic of neuroscience not to lead people astray, but to heal them.

Additional readings

Our study looking at reading and influencing thoughts with sham neuroimaging: Olson JA, Landry M, Appourchaux K, Raz A. Simulated thought insertion: influencing the sense of agency using deception and magic. Conscious Cogn 2016;43:11−26. Available from: https://doi.org/10.1016/j.concog.2016.04.010.

A related study exploring sham mind-to-mind communication with a similar device: Swiney L, Sousa P. When our thoughts are not our own: Investigating agency misattributions using the mind-to-mind paradigm. Conscious Cogn 2013;22(2):589−602. Available from: https://doi.org/10.1016/j.concog.2013.03.007.

Neuroplacebos: When healing is a no-brainer

16

Samuel Veissière

Neuroimaging has immense power. For the public, it seems to hold the promise of revealing the inner workings of brain, mind, and behavior. Neuroscientists are typically more modest. Through trial and error, they are hopeful that rigorous investigation will help elucidate basic mechanisms of cognition and disease. But do we really understand the extent of neuroimaging's magic sway on the public imagination?

Culturally, as the brain has largely replaced the soul, mind, or heart as the seat of personhood and behavior, the stories we tell ourselves about the invisible forces that regulate existence are more persuasive than ever. They are also bolstered by some of the most advanced medical technology ever devised. But what happens when these stories take on a life of their own? What happens when we leverage the power, not of neuroimaging technology itself, but of our culturally rooted *belief* in the power of such technology?

In a test to measure the physiological extent of the public's faith in neuroimaging, my colleagues and I have experimented with a novel application of these techniques: neuroplacebos. By relying on the trust individuals invest in neuroscience, and brain images in particular, we have induced surprisingly potent placebo effects in subjects suffering from a broad range of ailments. Indeed the public's faith in the authority of neuroimaging might just open up an avenue for the most potent culturally enhanced superplacebos ever devised.

We might greet the prospect of employing such neuroplacebos with enthusiasm. By the same token, the power of neuroimaging stories raises important questions about the ease with which we can bypass our critical faculties. What do we neuroimagers who tell those stories owe to the general public by way of honest disclosure? Perhaps more importantly, how do we avoid being seduced by the potency of our own technology and the stories we tell ourselves about it?

From built-in biases to mind—body regulation

Let's start with a quick primer on how placebos function more generally. In popular imagination, placebos are usually thought of as inert pills having no medical

Casting Light on the Dark Side of Brain Imaging. DOI: https://doi.org/10.1016/B978-0-12-816179-1.00016-5

properties and working through the power of belief alone. Because people expect them to be medicine, and because the priestly class of medicine is wrapped in such a halo of prestige, expectations do the heavy lifting of healing.

But placebos need not entail a pill. Sham surgeries with nothing more than an anesthesia procedure and a superficial cut-and-stitch ritual have been known to be very effective in the treatment of chronic pain.

Most recipes for placebo effects draw on well-established cognitive biases toward prestige and rarity, and in turn, on the conditioning of positive expectancies primed by social influences. Placebo effects are stronger, for instance, when the experimenters look like real doctors and when the settings look clinical. Treatments that seem expensive and hard to get work better than those that look cheap and easily accessible. Technologically elaborate placebos (such as sham surgeries) work better than pills.

Culture is embedded in this process in many general ways: for intuitions to be really strong, people must expect that enough people from their group also expect the same thing. As experiments undertaken with colleagues in McGill's Raz Lab have revealed, tapping into people's most deeply held cultural expectations provokes the strongest healing responses of all.

Medical magic

Once we've established the general conditions for effective placebos, we need to establish *which* contextual and cultural cues will best instantiate those conditions. Here we may rely on what Dr. Amir Raz has termed *neuroenchantment*. In a series of clever experiments Raz, a former professional magician and his researchers have found that even advanced students in psychology and neuroscience could be tricked into thinking that a crudely built sham brain scanner can produce improbable diagnostic and physiological effects. Exposed to fake brain technology built from a hairdresser's chair and discarded odds, participants had no trouble believing that the machine was reading their thoughts [1]. With a later, more realistic-looking (but equally fake) brain imaging machine, participants believed that the technology could not only read, but also influence their thoughts [2]; many reported an "unknown force" directing their thinking toward specific numbers (see Chapter 15).

Jay Olson, an experimental psychologist who, like Raz, first trained as a magician, finds that the sham scanner can even get participants to change their moral attitudes. The conclusion is clear: As decades of research in the science of decision-making have shown, humans are usually blind to context, prone to intuitive errors, and extraordinarily "receptive" instead of "prone" to influence by culture and prestige. On the other hand the same research reveals those processes as key to mind–body regulation. This fact carries consequences for a number of physiological responses that lie outside conscious control—including, it turns out, the body's ability to heal itself.

Neuroplacebos in practice

To see how all of this works in practice, let's take the case of one neuroplacebo success story. Matthew is a 9-year-old who suffered from chronic debilitating migraines. Six months before our initial experiment, he was primed by being told that he "might have a chance to be selected for a very expensive new cure" in which a very elaborate machine would "teach his brain how to heal itself and push out the pain of his headaches." Multiple family members and friends told the boy stories of this revolutionary new treatment, and he began asking when or if he would be selected for the project.

When the day finally came, everything from the hospital setting, the waiting room ritual, the large banners depicting cartoon brains and the word NEURO in light blue conspired to induce healing expectations. Clad in white coats and wielding clipboards, Olson and a female assistant walked little Matthew through a perfunctory medical interview before inviting him to lay in the mock-scanner. As he anxiously entered the noisy machine, he was told that "invisible gamma rays" would find the faulty connections in his brain and teach it to heal itself quicker and quicker. Matthew later confessed to his father that he had had a migraine before entering "Dr. Olson's room," and that the pain disappeared mere minutes after entering the machine. Over the next few weeks the frequency, longevity, and intensity of Matthew's migraines decreased by more than half.

In a second session, in which he felt more relaxed and eager to reenter the machine, Matthew was shown sham 3-D brain images rotating on a computer screen as pre- and posttreatment results. The first picture, representing his brain before treatment, was littered with red parts ostensibly showing where his pain originated. A second image, with radiating 3-D blue streaks, highlighted just "how well his brain had learned to heal itself." Four weeks after his second session, Matthew has not experienced a single migraine since.

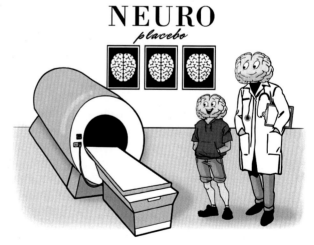

Our pilot experiments so far strongly suggest that the battery of healing effects that can be induced under hypnosis can be replicated with greater ease under accessory-assisted suggestion.

The power of symbols, rituals, accessories, and curated contexts—those that underlie *neuroenchantment* in particular—allows us to bypass costly induction methods and produce faster, stronger, longer healing responses.

The strange power of labeling "diseases" with brain images

In a subsequent study using the mock-scanner to help children with behavioral difficulties [3,4], we had initially planned to show children sham functional magnetic resonance imaging (fMRI) images and tell them that "their brain looks really good, and works very, very well." We would proceed to show them red and blue areas in pretty images, and tell them we had found "lots of activity in parts of their brain associated with being calm, focused, confident, and kind to others." After trying this procedure in pilot phases, we decided to drop the sham brain images due to an unexpected finding: the suggestive power of imaging was working *too well*.

After obtaining promising results with migraines, self-control, relaxation, and emotional regulation in pilot phases, we decided to make our procedure open-label—meaning that we would be transparent with the children and parents about our use of suggestion, and emphasize that all the healing effects they might notice would be caused by the children's own positive expectancies. We didn't want the children's symptoms to relapse after they found out about the placebo condition, and we didn't want them to associate all medical interventions with lies and deception. Above all, we wanted to help ingrain self-healing responses that could assist children in regaining a positive outlook on their life. Many of the parents in our study, as we discovered, didn't quite see it that way: they wanted us to comment on the brain images, and they wanted to know what was *wrong* with their children's brains.

We had briefed parents extensively on the phone before they gave us their informed consent and agreed to participate in our study. We had told them, in simple language, that the MRI was deactivated, that it could not read or influence brains, and that it was used as a placebo to help their child increase confidence and self-regulation. They had asked many questions about the procedure. They had heard us explain to their child, in even simpler language, that the machine was inert. Yet, after sham scanning sessions, many parents would repeatedly ask us to comment on pathological findings from the (sham) brain images. Two parents from the cohort repeated the question again in subsequent sessions after having been told again that the pictures were part of the placebo condition.

How to make sense of this strange finding?

One possible explanation comes foremost to mind. A saturation of prestige cues from the setting of our study had likely induced the caregivers' persisting blindness to our placebo condition despite our having briefed them. The study took place in the real brain imaging unit of a neurological hospital, replete with mandatory white coats, stethoscopes, and magnetic pass-operated sliding doors. The ongoing mental effort required to sustain the knowledge that everything about the study was fake amid such realistic décor must have been extraordinarily demanding.

That participants in a placebo study would revert to an automatic "real hospital schema" is understandable. That parents would frame their naïve questions about brain images as close-ended and negative ("what is *wrong* with my child's brain?," and not "did you find anything in the brain scan?") warrants critical investigation.

The culture of *neuroenchantment* goes beyond a world saturated with "brain breaks" in elementary schools, and an explosion of new "neuro"-disciplines from neuro-ethics and neuro-esthetics to neuro-economics and neuro-leadership. As the general public adopts the reductionist biochemical worldview of mainstream neuroscience and psychiatry such as that proposed by National Institute of Mental Health's RDoC [5], "neurochemical" and "faulty brain" folk explanations are increasingly being leveraged to account for such everyday processes as mood swings, affective fluctuations, and attentional shifts.

The immense rise in the diagnosis of Attention Deficit Disorders globally over the past decade [6] is a testament to that effect. The growing technological mediation of childhood, the increase in time spent with fast-paced devices, and the drastic decrease of unstructured play [7] have certainly led to a normalization of ever shorter attention spans, and in turn to broader expectations that children's attention spans are getting shorter. While elucidating the workings of attention and human behavior are likely to remain slow and mysterious processes, we as cognitive scientists must find better ways to convey these mysteries to the public. As it stands, we have trafficked in simplistic labels attached to pretty brain pictures that most often serve to frame negative expectations about what people can and cannot do.

Our experiments have taught me that inviting people to change their expectations can lead to immensely positive life transformations. I've also learned that expectations are strongly mediated by prestigious social influences, and that neuroscience provides the most salient and powerful of such influences in our society.

For scientists and laypeople alike, the negative effects of neuro-reductionism and the neuro-pathologization of everything have yet to be fully appreciated. Consider this chapter a modest call to neuroscientists, and an invitation to appreciate, then positively reframe, the strange power of their magic.

Additional readings

In this thought-provoking, myth-busting collection, Amir Raz, Irving Kirsch, Elizabeth
Loftus, and key scholars in the field of placebo studies tell us how social influences and
our expectations alone can produce drastic bodily responses in such domains as food,
mental illness and psychopharmacology, sex or false memories: Raz A, Harris C, editors. Placebo talks: modern perspectives on placebos in society. Oxford University
Press; 2016.

This far-reaching edited collection presents critical views from neuroscientists, philosophers,
psychiatrists, anthropologists, and cognitive scientists who reflect on the social biases,
cultural dimensions, and societal implications of neuroscience. Critical neuroscience is
also an invitation to transcend traditional skepticism, and explore novel ideas about
'how to be critical' in and about science: Choudhury S, Slaby J, editors. Critical neuroscience: a handbook of the social and cultural contexts of neuroscience. John Wiley &
Sons; 2016.

Brain imaging and artificial intelligence

Uri Maoz and Erik Linstead

Humans are generally fine with other humans policing them, managing their finances, driving them around, and making other critical decisions for them. This might be surprising as human decision-making is often irrational, if not biased [1]. It is also stochastic and inconsistent: faced with the same stimulus, humans sometimes make opposite choices. In addition, little is known about how decisions and actions are formulated in the brain. Even with brain imaging within the skull (intracranial) and inside the brain (intracortical), predicting simple human decisions from brain activity—such as which hand a person will use to press a button—remains difficult [2]. It is therefore all the more unclear how to mimic these neural processes using artificial systems.

Can we count on future forms of neuroimaging? Might these techniques one day lead to enough understanding of human decision-making to reproduce it artificially? After all, brain-imaging hardware is constantly improving. And great strides have been made in the analysis of neuroimaging in recent years, especially with regard to multivariate decoding, time-varying connectivity analysis, single-subject as well as large datasets analysis, together with commendable efforts at standardization and reproducibility [3,4].

What is more, these advances in neuroimaging have come in parallel with considerable advances in neurally inspired artificial intelligence (AI—though it is unclear to what extent neuroimaging will help us create human-like AI; see Chapter 1). A subfield of machine learning—termed *artificial neural-networks* (ANNs, also *deep learning*) because of its superficial structural resemblance to biological neural networks—has become especially successful of late. Fueled by a combination of specialized hardware, new algorithms, and the availability of large datasets, AI can now perform cognitive tasks that were previously deemed "exclusively human." Computers beat human world champions in the board game Go (in 2016), in Jeopardy (2011), and 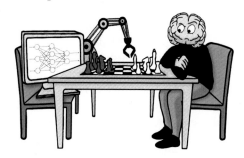 in Chess (in 1996). AI voice recognition rivals that of humans (even in noisy environments) and AI-based classification of photos into predetermined categories achieved accuracies similar to humans. Modern AI now also drives autonomous

Casting Light on the Dark Side of Brain Imaging. DOI: https://doi.org/10.1016/B978-0-12-816179-1.00017-7

cars, improves medical diagnosis, assists with financial decisions, and even cracks CAPTCHA images specifically constructed to be solvable by humans but not machines [5].

What does modern artificial intelligence look like?

Many people have begun to worry that the general-purpose AI of sci-fi is upon us, and that it will dethrone humans as the most intelligent beings on the planet—with the usual subsequent doomsday human enslavement of sci-fi lore. But general-purpose AI is neither here nor (likely) around the corner [5—7]—especially not one involving sentient, conscious, intentional robots. Again, humans understand too little about how the brain enables consciousness, volition, perception, and other high-level processing to reconstruct it in silicon [8].

But the doomsayers might just be barking up the wrong tree. Computers and robots have been replacing human labor for decades. Yet they have only recently learned to see (and, in particular, read), hear, and speak accurately enough to be useful. AI might therefore disrupt human lives other than by the physical enslavement of sci-fi lore [9]. That is partly because humans increasingly use AI as an aid for various types of decision-making—for example, in medicine and even construction [10]. But the bulk of the concern about nonmilitary applications of AI centers on the its increasing role in legal decision-making (bail, sentencing, parole, and predictive policing—e.g., the COMPAS system) and in financial risk-assessment (mortgages, credit scores, and loan approvals, as well as professional hiring and retention [11,12]). AI has a clear, direct, and potentially defining influence on the lives and future of people in these domains, yet few people understand how AI algorithms work.

The most successful branch of AI, ANNs, is implemented on computers. They are typically (though not always) composed of layers upon layers of units, termed *neurons* (although they are computational units, rather than biological material), that are each connected to neurons in the layer above. The strengths of these connections, or *weights*, are the free parameters that the ANN learns from the data. Such ANN models learn general rules from examples of the data. For instance given many pictures of dogs and cats, an ANN would learn what it is about the pictures that distinguishes cats from dogs (e.g., the shape of the ears, eyes, and whiskers; their relative positions; etc.) and be able to classify pictures that it had not previously seen. ANNs further learn increasingly abstract representation of the data in increasing layers of the network [13]. In the dog/cat example an ANN might represent local features—like eyes and whiskers—in the weights of lower layers and more-global features—like spatial relations among more-local features —in higher layers. Such models can be notoriously large with billions of free parameters over all the layers [14]. So, humans often cannot directly examine the weights to get a clear sense of how the ANN is manipulating the input. Researchers are aware of this problem and are attempting to make ANNs more interpretable to humans [15].

Some advantages of artificial neural networks over the human brain

These indirect manners of understanding complex AI models nevertheless leave some with concerns about algorithm-aided decision-making and certainly with autonomous AI making decisions. Note, though, that while we may not understand the specifics of the representation and decision rule that an ANN infers from the data, we do precisely know the formula determining each neuron's output from its input [14]. In contrast a complete computational model of single neurons in the human brain still eludes us. And there are hundreds of types of neurons in the human brain currently know that come in various shapes and biological specifications. We remain far from understanding each one fully, let alone from modeling their dynamics [16]. Additionally, controversy persists over how to model neural decision-making computationally, even with known neuronal models [17]. A second issue is that the activity of biological neurons, like human behavior, appears to be stochastic. So we cannot simply replay biological neuronal activity. Third, humans cannot easily rewire their biological neural networks and learn new rules. Thus a human driver who makes a mistake cannot replay the same exact scenario until they stop repeating that mistake and others like it.

Clear advantages of machine-learning algorithms that should receive more attention are the reproducibility of their results and the ease of rewiring them. While often complex and difficult to interpret, running these algorithm multiple times from a known initial state—or "replaying the algorithms"—on the same data produces identical results. Thus, for example, we could replay an error of a self-driving car until the range of inputs on which the car's algorithm fails is clearly delineated and corrected. Interestingly, humans generally do not extend the same level of trust to AI as they do to other humans—biased, irrational, and fallible as they might be.

From artificial neural networks to neuroimaging

Going back to neuroimaging, what we have learned about ANNs can help us better understand the limitations of future brain-imaging. Imagine that we were able to record the activity of every neuron in the human brain and had the computational capacity to analyze the petabytes of data that such activity would generate every second (complete science fiction at this point). And, with another leap of our imagination, say that we could model this huge, resulting neural network. Would we then know how the brain works?

First, biological factors other than neurons influence behavior: hormones, glial cells, and even our microbiome [18–20]. So, we would need to model their influence also, which we do not currently know how to do. Second, the type of access that we currently enjoy to ANNs is the one we are imagining we could have to biological neurons using future neuroimaging. What is more, these hypothetical, future models will likely mimic the biological neurons' intrinsic stochasticity, much more complex representation of individual neurons, and so on. So, they will be much more complex than current ANNs. And there is no reason to think that they would be any more interpretable than current ANNs, with which we are having such a hard time.

Completely reducing decisions to brain activity may therefore never be possible. Furthermore, even if we could somehow overcome all the obstacles above, this would still not let us rewire the brain in the same manner that we can rewire ANNs. Therefore baring future leaps beyond our current imagination, we can conclude that simply bigger and better neuroimaging will not be the silver bullet to building sci-fi-style machines with general AI. We simply do not know enough about how the brain works to create good models of human decision-making.

Conclusion

Greater incorporation of AI into human life will bring with it considerable change, producing winners and losers. So, the fear of AI may simply be fear of the new and unknown. Or it could be a form of speciesism, a combination of the above, or something else altogether [21]. But AI appears to be here to stay. And, as these ANNs become increasingly large and complex, the understanding we gain about their function, composition, and limitations might also help us better understand some aspects of the workings of the human brain [8]. For example, neuroscientists are looking forward to future neuroimaging techniques that would let them record ever-larger brain networks. But what we have learned about humans' inability to make out how the weights of complex ANNs translate into their impressive performance on nontrivial cognitive tasks, suggests limitations on the human ability to understand such future, large-scale recordings. So, while AI began by borrowing concepts and models from neuroscience, current and future AI might return the favor by helping neuroscientists better understand the brain as well as recognize the limitations of human understanding of the brain.

Additional readings

A paper highlighting past, current, and future shared themes between neuroscience and AI: Hassabis D, Kumaran D, Summerfield C, Botvinick M. Neuroscience-inspired artificial intelligence. Neuron 2017;95(2):245−58.

A good, though technical, book about the modern theory of ANNs: Goodfellow I, Bengio Y, Courville A. Deep learning. Cambridge, MA: The MIT Press; 2016. 775 pp.

An ethical discussion about whether legal personhood should be conferred on AI agents: Bryson JJ, Diamantis ME, Grant TD. Of, for, and by the people: the legal lacuna of synthetic persons. Artif Intell Law 2017;25(3):273−91.

An interesting report on the state of AI in 2017—measures of performance in some key cognitive tasks, including comparisons to human performance; academic- and business-related activity; expert forum; and so on: <http://www.aiindex.org/>.

Section V

Can we train the brain better?

Noninvasive brain stimulation: When the hype transcends the evidence

18

Jared Cooney Horvath

Nearly every major newspaper [1], magazine [2], website [3], radio program [4], and news show [5] has made the proclamation: the future is here!

In this future, people are using magnetic fields and electric currents to zap their brains and transcend the boundaries of typical human performance. Olympic athletes are strapping batteries to their head in order to run faster and jump higher. Soldiers are pulsing magnetic waves through their skull in order to sharpen focus and maintain vigilance. Students are pouring electrons into their brains to boost memory and hasten learning.

Here's the best part: although this all might feel like some science-fiction-induced delirium, it is based on over 30-years of laboratory-based, peer-reviewed, tax-payer-funded scientific research. In fact, since 1985, well over 10,000 scientific articles have been published expounding the ability of these noninvasive brain stimulation tools to impact and improve brain function.

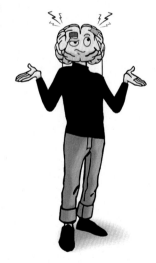

What are you waiting for? You can jump online *today* and buy some of these devices *right now* to turn yourself into the super-human you've always wanted to be (prices range from $50 for basic models up to $10,000 for research-grade machines).

The future is here!

...not so fast.

Over the last couple of years, a number of large-scale reviews, analyses, and studies have revealed that these machines may not actually be doing what they claim. In fact, mounting evidence suggests that these devices are *not* improving memory, learning, performance, mood, or anything else for that matter [6−14]. In fact, there is data to suggest that some of these devices do not even impact the brain, let alone change its function for the better [15].

A quick primer

Noninvasive brain stimulation devices typically come in two unique flavors: magnetic and electric.

The primary *magnetic* stimulation device is called repetitive transcranial magnetic brain stimulation (rTMS). This machine activates regions of the brain and (theoretically) alters their function for a prolonged period of time by sending long chains of rapidly fluctuating magnetic fields through the skull. Within the laboratory, rTMS can be utilized to map various brain functions while, within the clinic, it can be utilized as a treatment for specific forms of medication-resistant depression.

The primary *electric* stimulation device is called transcranial direct current stimulation (tDCS). This machine sends very weak electric currents across the scalp which (theoretically) enter the head and change the reactivity of different brain regions. Unlike rTMS, which force-fires neurons within the brain, tDCS simply makes neurons more or less *likely* to fire: there is no direct brain activation.

With regards to the enhancement potential of rTMS, the jury is still out. A number of studies have reported positive results, but there is a marked lack of meta-analyses and critical reviews that explore the impact of this tool in healthy (as opposed to clinical) populations. With regards to the enhancement potential of tDCS, despite there being hundreds of papers reporting positive results, a number of detailed reviews suggest this tool does not, in fact, alter brain function and likely has little-to-no impact on cognition. As such, the remainder of this chapter will focus on evidence obtained utilizing tDCS—however, the themes outlined throughout apply to all forms of noninvasive brain stimulation.

So, how did we get here? How did so many people put so much time and effort into building a bridge that appears to be leading nowhere?

The problem lies in "generality."

General versus specific findings

When discussing their work, most researchers necessarily speak in generalities; they highlight *major* findings and avoid drilling down into nuanced *specifics* so as to not confuse or bore listeners. Although this practice makes science and research more accessible to lay audiences, it is the breeding ground of *hype* and can lead even the most astute of minds to mistake smoke-and-mirrors for reality.

Here's a simple hypothetical example of how this error happens.

Imagine three different research papers all claim a certain brain stimulation device can improve your golf swing. Taken together, this sounds incredible! Three *different* scientists from three *different* labs running three *different* studies all saying the *same exact* thing—take my money!

Here's where things get tricky. A golf swing is not a "single" skill: rather, it's a broad term that encompasses many specific subskills. For instance, a golf swing involves speed, strength, and accuracy (to name just three).

Now, let's drill down and explore the specifics of each of these three studies. It turns out, study #1 improved swing *speed*, but had no impact on strength or accuracy; study #2 improved swing *strength*, but had no impact on speed or accuracy; and study #3 improved swing *accuracy*, but had no impact on speed or strength.

Importantly, when I say a study had "no impact" on certain skills, I do not mean that these skills were never examined (*absence of evidence*); I mean that these skills were actively measured and showed no change in response to brain stimulation (*evidence of absence*).

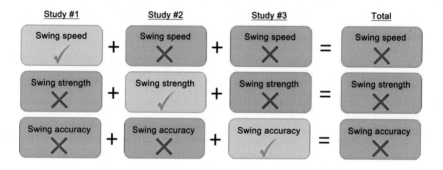

Do you see the problem here?

Speaking generally, these three studies all appear to be telling the same story: namely, that this device can improve your golf swing. This claim is not a lie (seeing as each study *did* find an improvement on a particular aspect of the golf swing), it is simply general.

However, speaking specifically, there is *twice as much evidence* suggesting this device actually has no impact on swing speed, strength, or accuracy. In other words, this device likely *will not* improve your golf swing.

Uh-oh!

This is the issue with noninvasive brain stimulation in a nut-shell. When speaking generally, there are reams of studies that suggest these devices can improve memory, intelligence, learning, performance, etc. This all sounds great...until you ask "What specifically do you mean by memory?"

Once we dive into the specifics, everything disappears. As earlier, each study typically shows improvement on a *specific* subskill while showing no change in a number of other subskills (remember: each of these subskills will be measured and reported within each study). Unfortunately, the specific subskill to show improvement differs between each study. This is why, as noted earlier, many large-scale reviews show no impact from brain stimulation [6−15]. At the general level (e.g., "memory"), dozens of studies show a positive effect. However, at the specific level (e.g., "accuracy of recognition memory" vs "speed of recognition memory"), everything cancels out, there is *far* more evidence suggesting no impact from brain stimulation, and, we're left grasping at smoke.

All aboard the hype-train

The fact that the popular press is picking up on and promoting brain stimulation to the masses is one of the greatest examples of the hype outstripping evidence today.

Don't get me wrong. I am not blaming the press or consumers for this hype. In this instance, the hype stems from scientists attempting to engage the public and get them excited about the possibilities of research. This desire is completely understandable...though, the execution has led us astray.

So, what can we learn from all of this?

Although there are dozens of lessons researchers can glean (*the difficulty of public science communication, the importance of robust research, the danger of overly simplifying abstracts, etc.*), I reckon there are four take-homes that transcend the laboratory and are important for researchers, journalists, consumers, and the lay public to consider.

1. In order for a drug or device to be useful, we must clearly define and report *who* will (and will not) benefit. It is not enough to say "This will work for some people" and never clarify who.
   Unfortunately, no one is yet certain who will (and won't) respond to brain stimulation. Which leads us to...

2. In order for a drug or device to be useful, we must clearly define and report *when* benefits will (and will not) occur. It's not enough to say "This will work some of the time" and never clarify when.
   Unfortunately, brain stimulation research reveals that the same person may respond positively one day, negatively the next day, and have no response the third day [16–19]. Importantly, there is no clear way to predict under what circumstance a person will respond in a particular way. This means no one is yet certain when these devices will (and won't) work as desired. Which leads us to...

3. In order for a drug or device to be useful, we must clearly define and report the *specific skills* that will (and will not) benefit. It is not enough to say "This device will make you smarter" and never clarify what is meant by "smarter."
   Unfortunately, no one is yet certain what specific aspects of thinking different brain stimulation devices will (and won't) impact. Which leads us to...

4. In order for a drug or device to be useful, it must be better than freely available techniques and methods.
   Unfortunately, there is no concrete (or compelling) evidence that brain stimulation can generate predictable, reliable, or significant effects. Conversely, there is a wealth of evidence demonstrating that methods like distributed practice, interleaving, direct instruction, and deliberate practice can predictably, reliably, and significantly boost learning, memory, skill performance, etc. [20].

If we do not know *who* brain stimulation will work for, *when* it will work, *how* it will work, or even *if* it will work better than traditional learning and training practices...perhaps this emerging technology is not quite ready for prime time.

Additional readings

An easy to read review that outlines the important issues (and shortcomings) of noninvasive brain stimulation research utilizing tDCS: Horvath JC, Carter O, Forte JD. Transcranial direct current stimulation: five important issues we aren't discussing (but probably should be). Front Syst Neurosci 2014;8.

A great critical introduction to varied methods of noninvasive brain stimulation, their potential in research and treatment, and the pit-falls in research conducted to date: Parkin BL, Ekhtiari H, Walsh VF. Non-invasive human brain stimulation in cognitive neuroscience: a primer. Neuron 2015;87(5):932−45.

Another easy to read review outlining the peaks and perils of tDCS research: Berryhill ME, Peterson DJ, Jones KT, Stephens JA. Hits and misses: leveraging tDCS to advance cognitive research. Front Psychol 2014;5.

Neurofeedback: An inside perspective

Jimmy Ghaziri and Robert T. Thibault

How much would you pay to improve your brain? What if you had problems of attention, depression, or anxiety—would you pay even more to rewire your brain and overcome your condition? For a few thousand dollars, many brain-training practitioners claim to provide this service. Using a technique called *neurofeedback*, they present individuals with a live feed of their own brain activity. By watching our brain, neurofeedback advocates argue that we can learn to regulate its activity and, in turn, control our behavior. The relevant data, however, reveal a more nuanced story. One of placebos.

In this chapter, we focus on the most popular neurofeedback modality and the only one applied clinically: electroencephalography neurofeedback, or simply EEG-nf. Our perspective comes from the angle of a former neurofeedback coach, and current neuroscientist (Ghaziri), and a cognitive neuroscientist who has extensively reviewed the EEG-nf literature (Thibault). Together, we argue that EEG-nf may help improve some conditions, but, at least in the way it is currently applied, this technique relies almost exclusively on placebo effects and psychoeducation (providing support and information to help people cope with their condition).

On the surface, EEG-nf looks like an advanced biomedical therapy. Practitioners sit patients down, apply electrodes to their scalp, and provide a simple auditory and/or visual cue to let participants know when their brain is "performing well." Depending on the patient's condition, positive feedback will stem from different brainwave frequencies. In psychological terms, EEG-nf uses operant conditioning to reward and train-specific brainwave patterns. Patients generally train for 30–60 minutes at a time and often return for up to 40 sessions. Where EEG-nf diverges most from standard-of-care biomedicine is in the subpar research on which it rests.

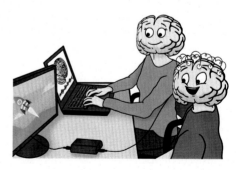

Although over 3000 research publications discuss EEG-nf, only 11 experiments meet the standard of clinical research: double-blind and placebo-controlled. In the

Casting Light on the Dark Side of Brain Imaging. DOI: https://doi.org/10.1016/B978-0-12-816179-1.00019-0

case of EEG-nf, a proper placebo control entails a "sham" feedback signal, often taken from the recordings of a previous participant [1]. Only one of these 11 studies, which aimed to rehabilitate stroke patients, showed a superiority of genuine over sham neurofeedback in terms of behavioral outcomes. Most of the other 10 experiments attempted to improve attention deficit hyperactivity disorder (ADHD) and demonstrated equivalent improvement between the experimental and control groups. Somewhat counterintuitively, the United States Food and Drug Administration (FDA) allows neurofeedback devices. Yet, only to promote relaxation. The FDA considers all other uses of neurofeedback as "off-label." Even then, the FDA never "approved" EEG-nf. Instead, EEG-nf squeezed through a grandfather loophole where any device in use prior to 1976 (which EEG-nf was) were allowed to continue being sold. Although regulatory agencies only accept EEG-nf for very narrow purposes, practitioners attempt to treat a wide range of conditions.

In my (Ghaziri's) 5 years of coaching under the supervision of a neuropsychologist, we used neurofeedback to help patients suffering from ADHD, anxiety, autism spectrum disorder, depression, tinnitus (ringing in the ears), headaches, traumatic brain injury, and epilepsy; as well as for general cognitive enhancement in healthy individuals. Patients with ADHD, anxiety, and depression seemed to show the most improvement. Although it remains difficult to identify what exactly helped patients in this clinical setting (owing to the lack of a control group). A positive relationship between practitioner and patient, the general benefits of cognitive training, and high levels of motivation seemed to go a long way. For anxiety in particular, patients I saw seemed to use the feedback as a cue to focus on their breathing and remain mindful of their mental state. If they felt anxious and tense, the feedback would alter—but even then, the electrical activity from muscles, rather than directly from the brain, may have driven this change (see Chapter 7). In many cases the benefits I observed seemed to rest largely on the coaching framework, mainly by reassuring the patients and providing tips for how to relax, and less on viewing one's own brainwaves. Robust studies back up this point and find that EEG-nf seems to improve some conditions, but independently of the feedback patients receive [2].

The literature on other conditions, such as tinnitus and epilepsy, suggests that EEG-nf may work, but the findings often come from experiments with few participants (see Chapter 12), no control group, and a body of evidence that may suffer from publication bias that sways the evidence in favor of EEG-nf. Thus for some patients where no other treatment seems to work, EEG-nf offers some hope as a last resort regardless of how strong the base of evidence.

Instead of focusing on behavior, some EEG-nf practitioners seem more interested in normalizing brainwaves. In a method termed quantitative EEG, or simply qEEG, these practitioners often deem neurofeedback successful when, after training, the brainwaves of patients more closely match an average profile derived from a database of scans taken from healthy individuals. And yet, idolizing "normal" brainwave patterns is like arguing that people should all strive to be the same "optimal" height—even if that means stretching some people and squishing others. The shape and size of the human brain and skull varies substantially between individuals. Even if two brains produced the same activity, the signal would look different by the time it reaches the EEG sensors placed on the scalp. Moreover, qEEG results are widely heterogeneous both between individuals and within single individuals at different time points. Numerous factors influence the qEEG including how you slept last night, whether you're having a good day, and if you drank coffee before the recording. When looking at the most comprehensive list of publications that specifically trained qEEG patterns, we find that 95% of the authors either practice this technique privately or sell the equipment to do so [3].

Rather than create "normal" brain activity, EEG-nf primarily aims to train positive behaviors that generalize into everyday life. In my own study, we found that EEG-nf alters the brain as measured by structural magnetic resonance imaging (MRI); however, we found poor behavioral differences between participants given genuine versus sham feedback [4]. While some EEG-nf advocates may argue that our study proves that EEG-nf entails measurable benefits above and beyond placebo effects, in terms of behavioral benefits it suggests the opposite, especially considering that the study does not meet the standard of clinical research (e.g., double-blind and sufficient sample size).

As neuroscientists, we must keep a critical eye on the literature. The lack of standard protocols is the weakest link of neurofeedback. Indeed, research reports rarely described the protocol used in full detail. Some clinicians seem to simply place their patients in front of a screen displaying neurofeedback for a half hour and hope that everything fixes itself. Other practitioners continuously interact with their patients throughout training. Some tailor the feedback to each patient. Others present standardized feedback. We imagine that regardless of why patients improve (via specific EEG-nf-related mechanisms or placebo effects), more interaction would help amplify positive treatment outcomes. Encouragement seems to help patients maintain a minimum level of effort that allows them to reap benefits. Hence, EEG-nf seems to be mostly a mindfulness training technique that would require a certain level of metacognition and self-regulation and uses neurotechnology to maximize participant motivation. In support of this point, meta-analyses show that deliberate practice, rather than other more general processes, accounts for only a small percentage of performance capacity across a number of domains such as playing video games (28%), learning a musical instrument (21%), and practicing a sport (18%) [5]).

This conclusion is worrisome when we consider the cost of EEG-nf and the population that seeks this treatment. They are often vulnerable, have exhausted many other treatment options, and decide to place their final hopes (and money) on up to 40 sessions of EEG-nf. With its current price tag, and the seeming equivalence between genuine and sham feedback, it should be practiced with some caution.

We do, however, maintain interest in the use of neurofeedback as a tool to control brain—computer interfaces (Chapter 4) and in research to better understand the relation between brain and behavior (Chapter 3). These fields come with a distinct literature and separate set of evidence compared to that surrounding EEG-nf. We also remain hopeful that other advancements in neurofeedback, such as combining fMRI-nf with machine-learning algorithms [6], will develop into fruitful treatments.

In a word, EEG-nf has yet to reach the status of evidence-based medicine. Robust experiments show an equivalence between genuine and sham EEG-nf. Nonetheless, EEG-nf practitioners continue to forge ahead while shying away from discussing the glaring caveats.

Additional readings

A popular-style and critical blog post on EEG-nf written by a buster of brain myths: <https://www.psychologytoday.com/blog/brain-myths/201302/read-paying-100s-neu-rofeedback-therapy-0>.

A succinct academic letter that highlights the peculiar climate surrounding EEG-nf research and practice: Thibault RT, Lifshitz M, Raz A. The climate of neurofeedback: Scientific rigour and the perils of ideology. Brain 2018;141(2):e11. Available from: http://doi.org/10.1093/brain/awx330.

A thorough and historical review of the most common neurofeedback modalities: Thibault RT, Lifshitz M, Birbaumer N, Raz A. Neurofeedback, self-regulation, and brain imaging: clinical science and fad in the service of mental disorders. Psychother Psychosomat 2015;84(4):193–207. Available from: https://doi.org/10.1159/000371714.

The (dis)enchantment of brain-training games

20

Sheida Rabipour

Imagine your favorite computer game—perhaps a stealthy mission to fight bad guys, a race through a tactical obstacle course, a mind-bending puzzle, or a popular team sport. Imagine losing yourself in guilt-free bliss, knowing that your virtual world of choice is also good for your brain, your mind, and even your overall health.

Few scientific fields have generated as much public intrigue and controversy as brain training. From simple brainteasers to wearable devices that monitor or stimulate brain activity, brain-training programs have enchanted researchers, clinicians, and consumers with the promise of reengineering the brain to increase productivity, rehabilitate injury, and reverse disease. Perhaps most prominent are computerized or virtual reality games advertised to enhance the brain through repeated practice of a mentally demanding task. The ability to peer inside the living, working brain through neuroimaging techniques has taught us that our daily activities do, indeed, change the way our brain looks and functions. As a result, hundreds of programs—including the famed *BrainHQ, Cogmed, Cognifit, Lumosity*, and countless emerging products—fuel a billion-dollar industry [1] that shows no sign of abating. Amid all the hype, the fundamental question remains: does brain training really work? This lingering debate highlights the darker side of brain training where, even among experts, there is no consensus on the practical benefits of brain games (for discussion of other types of neuroenhancement, see Chapters 18 and 19). And as the evidence accumulates, so does the skepticism

The appeal of brain training is unequivocal. Many of us know the pain of seeing a loved one slip away into dementia or lose the ability to think and act independently following injury. Few people, if any, would turn down the opportunity to be a little more mentally sharp, creative, or productive. Mainstream society is competitive; we live in a culture that often applauds long work hours over personal life. Many of us feel like we need an edge. For those born without the natural abilities or social privileges of others, brain training offers a possible method of "catching up." Outside the domain of personal development, even the most skeptical of academics cannot deny the potential of various techniques to

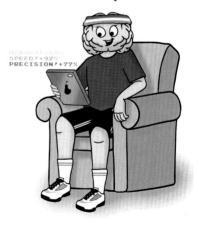

Casting Light on the Dark Side of Brain Imaging. DOI: https://doi.org/10.1016/B978-0-12-816179-1.00020-7

enlighten us about the mechanisms of change in the brain and body. Better yet, all this might be possible noninvasively, without requiring the surgeon's knife or the pharmacist's potion. Such enlightenment could result from the simple act of playing a game or slapping on some headgear, and often from the comfort and privacy of home. From all perspectives, brain training is a tantalizing prospect. But, as is often the case, if something seems too good to be true, it probably is.

Recent history has toppled brain training from its pedestal, its reputation diminished by numerous limitations and, in some cases, by outright fraud. Programs advertised to improve memory, focus, and efficiency in daily activities have rarely delivered on their promises. Some available products have no scientific evidence supporting them. Companies have received backlash, even federal lawsuits, for deceptive marketing using unfounded claims that prey on concerns surrounding aging and rehabilitation. For example, ads for *Lumosity* once dominated the media with claims of helping users remember names and birthdates, concentrate better, think faster, and "build a better brain [...] in a way that just feels like games." With millions of subscribers and the implication that their games could even stave off cognitive decline, *Lumosity*, like many other programs who made such claims, was thriving. But in early 2016 the Federal Trade Commission (FTC) of the United States filed a complaint against the creators of *Lumosity* for "deceiv[ing] consumers with unfounded claims that *Lumosity* games can help users perform better at work and in school, and reduce or delay cognitive impairment associated with age and other serious health conditions," costing the company $2 million in settlements out of a pending $50 million fine [2]. The story of *Lumosity*, perhaps the most striking, is unfortunately not unique. In 2015 the FTC filed a similar complaint against the makers of *Jungle Rangers*, a program claiming to improve memory, attention, behavior, and school performance in children. These cases have served as cautionary tales to all brain-training companies who overstate the benefits of their products without substantiated scientific evidence.

Brain training draws on the allure of neuroplasticity and the vibrant brain images captured by neuroimaging techniques. Although once unfathomable [3], we now know that the brain's many neurons continuously change in response to our daily experiences and can grow more abundant through the process of neuroplasticity. The malleability of the brain is reflected in our behavior, and in our ability to adapt to our surroundings and learn to thrive in different settings. We experience this process throughout life, as we learn to handle tools (e.g., a fork and knife to eat, a pencil or keyboard to communicate) and master musical instruments, sports, or other skills. Brain imaging techniques have confirmed this phenomenon, demonstrating links between activity in particular brain areas or networks and the performance of specific tasks.

The discovery of neuroplasticity and the invention of brain imaging heralded an exciting era of possibility in brain science. Many jumped on the idea of leveraging the dynamics of neuroplasticity to deliberately shape performance by engaging in these types of activities, using neuroplasticity as a blanket justification for unsupported claims. Thus, the brain-training industry—and controversy—was born.

In the early days of brain training, excitement seemed warranted. In both children and adults, training with computer games targeting specific mental skills seemed to improve capacities such as attention, memory, and information processing, as well as the symptoms of common behavioral disorders [4−6]. As an educational module, programs focusing on structured play or listening skills appeared to improve emotional and social skills [7], perception of tones and literacy [8], and other mental capacities crucial to scholastic achievement [9]. Beyond improvements in behavior and performance, researchers found training-related changes in the brain, both when people performed a challenging task and at rest [10]. For example, studies showed different patterns of brain activity in people who frequently played video games compared to nongamers [11], and in people who engaged in just a few hours of mindfulness meditation training [12]. These changes were alleged to underlie improvements in the control of attention. Companies, and some researchers, used such brain scans as objective proof that brain training works, without necessarily considering how sustainable these changes might be or whether other activities could induce comparable improvements. Brain training came to be viewed—and advertised—as a potential panacea for age-related pathology, psychiatric illness, and brain injury.

The early evidence that launched brain training onto its flourishing commercial trajectory has been insufficient to justify its continued success. Company websites often draw on handpicked testimonials or unrepresentative case studies to support the effectiveness of their products. The greatest evidence for brain training comes from flawed research using inappropriate methodology. Too often, small improvements in a specific lab environment have been inaccurately exaggerated into headlines hailing brain training as a cure for memory loss or distractibility, with colorful brain images to give the appearance of credibility. Even the more rigorous studies are inconsistent in choosing the type of people they study (e.g., developing children, healthy young adults, clinical populations, or those beginning to feel the mental toll of aging) as well as the tools they use to measure outcomes. Gauging the scientific literature on brain training is not an easy feat.

Moreover, scientists evaluating programs have rarely taken into account individual factors that could shape outcomes. For example, in a climate of highly advertised products and vivid debates, brain-training studies have typically failed to consider how people's expectations of the effectiveness of a program might affect the program's outcomes. In other words, a program may seem beneficial simply because people believe they will improve certain abilities, leading them to invest more time and effort engaging in a particular activity. The converse is true as well: if people don't expect an activity to enhance some aspect of their life, they are unlikely to engage with it productively enough to perceive any improvement. How can we evaluate programs without considering all the factors that influence training?

The challenges of evaluating brain training become even greater when considering the variability between existing programs. Brain training represents a wide category of products that fit into the larger context of mental fitness. In addition to computerized, targeted mental exercises, the field has grown to encompass digital technologies (e.g., virtual and augmented reality video games) and holistic lifestyle habits (e.g., mindfulness meditation), as well as more traditional forms of training typically restricted to therapeutic interventions (e.g., strategy training). Individual programs often borrow bits and pieces of other exercises, merging computer games with technology to monitor one's own brain activity (e.g., neurofeedback) or to deliver weak electric currents to the surface of the scalp (e.g., transcranial electrical stimulation), purported to accelerate learning and performance gains. The nature of different types of training as well as the context in which they are applied make it difficult to compare programs and determine whether support or criticism for one program applies to another.

The case of brain training highlights the pitfalls of premature commercialization before establishing effectiveness and practical societal value. For brain training to graduate beyond preliminary support, more studies will have to adopt the gold standard of randomizing large samples, using control groups that are matched in variables unrelated to the subject of study (e.g., age, education, socioeconomic background), and accounting for factors known to influence the outcomes of behavioral interventions. Objective tools such as brain imaging can serve as a powerful ally to a well-designed study. To be most worthwhile, brain-training programs should lead to broad improvements that generalize to contexts outside the lab setting. The problem, however, is that many approaches do the opposite: programs may train your ability to remember a set of objects while playing a game, and may even help you remember a slightly different sequence a few minutes later, but they are less likely to help you memorize your grocery list or remember where you left those darned keys.

Despite the pitfalls of brain training, even researchers have a hard time dismissing the enterprise. In 2014, hundreds of prominent and respected academics divided themselves into two seemingly opposing camps, signing a statement either supporting [13] or refuting [14] the effectiveness of brain training. The statements nevertheless came to the same general conclusion: although brain-training programs have largely over-promised and under-delivered, the endeavor may still prove valuable with more rigorous research.

Context is key when considering the value of brain training. For example, high-functioning people may benefit more from complex game-based software that combines multiple types of tasks and requires adaptive problem-solving compared to simpler or more specifically targeted exercises, which may work best for the rehabilitation of functions lost as a result of injury or disease. Asking whether brain training "works" is therefore a flawed and, to a certain extent, meaningless question. Arguably, the better question is whether a particular program can help achieve an overarching goal. In other words: what kind of practice or technique might benefit a particular type of person in a given circumstance?

The decision to pursue brain training is personal. Computer games may add little value if you're already concerned about declining memory or focus and have made other changes in your lifestyle—eating better, exercising more, seeking new and challenging reading material, perhaps even doing some of your own research on brain health. Similarly, if your daily activities rely heavily on technology, chances are that 15 minutes of web-based brainteasers will do little more to challenge your mental faculties. Conversely, if a technology is new to you, or if you feel isolated with scarce opportunity for socializing, digital programs may provide some of the mental stimulation you are lacking, and may further provide an opportunity to connect with other players or access a coach virtually.

Those enamored with brain training often forget that we already shape our mental and physical health in an important way. Through education, we enhance our capacity to think critically and draw associations to solve new problems; through repeated practice, we enhance our memory, perhaps to learn a new skill or memorize lengthy text; through nutritional diet and constructive lifestyle habits, we optimize our wellbeing and performance in daily activities. Brain scans have further shown that certain activities—e.g., meditating, navigating a complex terrain, learning to juggle or play a musical instrument, and playing video games—may alter brain structure and function, even in adulthood. What many consumers don't necessarily realize is that such changes occur naturally—a vulnerability that many companies bank on.

New brain-training approaches are constantly emerging, but many of them remain experimental and the evidence for their effectiveness is inconclusive. Despite the initial hype and commercial success of brain training, recent evidence calls for greater scrutiny of existing modules and a shift in perspectives regarding the applicability of brain training. Yet the need for greater scrutiny hardly means we should abandon our quest for tools and techniques that help optimize our thought and behavior. The past encourages us to exercise caution in our enchantment, without letting it wane into disillusionment.

Additional readings

An overview of brain training approaches and applications in research, medicine, education, parenting, and industry: Rabipour S, Raz A. Training the brain: fact and fad in cognitive and behavioral remediation. Brain Cogn 2012;79:159−79. Available from: https://doi.org/10.1016/j.bandc.2012.02.006.

A study of people's expectations of brain training, and why they matter: Rabipour S, Andringa R, Boot WR, Davidson PSR. What do people expect of cognitive enhancement? J Cogn Enhance 2017;1−8. Available from: https://doi.org/10.1007/s41465-017-0050-3.

A reader-friendly, academic review of physical and cognitive enhancement in aging: Rabipour S, Miller D, Taler V, Messier C, Davidson PSR. Handbook of gerontology research methods: understanding successful aging. Routledge; 2017.

An academic review and critique of brain training methods in science: Simons DJ, et al. Do "brain-training" programs work? Psychol Sci Public Interest 2016;17:103−86. Available from: https://doi.org/10.1177/1529100616661983.

What's wrong with "the mindful brain"? Moving past a neurocentric view of meditation

21

Michael Lifshitz and Evan Thompson

Riding a growing wave of scientific data, mindfulness meditation has found its way to the forefront of popular culture. Mindfulness practices appeal to a wide spectrum of society, from stressed out office workers and college students to stock traders, doctors, government officials, and even infantry soldiers. These practices have come a long way from their humble beginnings at the outskirts of ancient Indian society. Mindfulness has emerged as a major force in global culture—enshrined in national medical guidelines, showcased on trendwatcher lists, and raking in over a billion dollars in profit each year [1].

The growing mindfulness hype revolves around a particular view of mindfulness meditation as a kind of brain training [2]. At the heart of this trend lies a simple idea with apparently massive appeal: practicing meditation, we are told, literally rewires your brain [3]. It's a catchy idea: train your mind, change your brain [4]. But this idea has its problems, both empirical (as to the strength of the available evidence) and conceptual (as to whether it even makes sense to think of meditation in these terms).

In this chapter, we argue that the neurocentric view of mindfulness meditation, a perspective we call "the mindful brain," is a simplistic take on what meditation is and how it works. Contrary to the neurocentic view, we see meditation as a deeply social, and fundamentally embodied collection of practices. If we reduce meditative practices to a set of brain patterns, we miss the richness of how these practices work and ignore much of what they have to teach us about human experience [5].

The appeal of the mindful brain

In today's language, mindfulness is understood as a state, or trainable skill, of paying attention in a particular way. To be mindful is to become aware of the ongoing stream of present-moment experience with an attitude of curiosity and acceptance. According to this popular understanding, mindfulness is about noticing what's going on with your thoughts, your body, and your emotions—taking stock of the

Casting Light on the Dark Side of Brain Imaging. DOI: https://doi.org/10.1016/B978-0-12-816179-1.00021-9

subtle nuances of lived experience that we tend to gloss over in our busy lives. By training particular networks in our brains, we can learn to pay attention in this mindful way. It's not hard to see why this idea appeals to our contemporary sensibilities. We live in a wired world that relentlessly assaults us with complexity. Mindfulness seems to offer private access to a simpler mode of consciousness. It can give us a sense of control over our inner lives. The popular, yet misguided, idea that mindfulness resides in the brain suggests that the key to our happiness, peace, and productivity lies within. By controlling our brain, we take control of our own subjective well-being.

If there's one thing our contemporary culture values more than individual self-determination, it's tangible results. We put our faith in what we can measure. The concept of the *mindful brain* suggests that practicing mindfulness meditation really *does* something—something physical, concrete. The proof, apparently, is in the brain pudding. Studies suggest that Buddhist monks (the "Olympic athletes" of meditation) have thicker brains in all the right places, and that even busy westerners can thicken their brains after just a few weeks of daily meditation [6]. The implication is clear: if we are willing to meditate just a few minutes per day, we too can rewire our brains to gain more awareness and control over our own minds—to become happier, more productive, and more peaceful on the inside.

It's appealing to think that we might identify a specific brain signature of the mindful state. Then we might optimize meditation training to achieve that state more quickly and easily. We could skip all the fluff that has tended to come along with meditation (the religious cosmology, the moral doctrines, the bells, and robes) and focus on what some people take to be the real essence: strengthening the brain's attention networks to achieve nonjudgmental awareness of our own experience. Ostensibly, this optimized neuro-mindfulness approach will get us the results we want, and fast. Since the advent of the *mindful brain*, finding inner peace has never been easier. These days, you don't even need to seek out a meditation teacher or community—you can just download a mindfulness app or strap on a brain-sensing headband to ramp up your brainwaves. For a low cost, and just a few minutes of your time, you too can have your own mindful brain.

Limitations of the mindful brain

The finding that meditation changes your brain is often taken as a kind of proof that meditation really *works*. The tacit understanding seems to be that documenting the effects of meditation on the physical tissue of the brain makes these effects more substantial and reliable, more trustworthy—more *real*. But all mental activity is presumably reflected at the level of brain function, so it's hardly surprising that a change in mental behavior corresponds to a change in the brain. Any repetitive activity you do is likely to leave lasting traces on your brain. Learning to play an instrument, acquiring a second language, playing video games, or even staring at lines on a screen—all of these activities have been shown to mold the brain.

Meditation is far from unique in this regard, so it makes little sense to appeal to the idea that mindfulness practice changes your brain as a way of proving that it really has effects. If a practice changes subjective experience, it almost certainly changes the brain.

What remains less obvious, however, is whether current brain imaging methods can accurately pick up and make sense of the changes in the brain brought about by practices such as mindfulness meditation. The scientific evidence that meditative practices leave lasting positive imprints on the brain remains tentative [2]. For one thing, much of the available evidence relies on correlation, not causation. The majority of studies investigating meditation-induced neuroplasticity compare long-term meditators to novices. From these studies alone, we cannot ascertain whether the observed brain differences are really due to the practice of meditation or simply reflect a preexisting difference between the groups. Perhaps people with thicker brains in certain regions are just more likely to take up the practice of meditation and stick to it.

Neuroscientists who study meditation are well aware of the limitations of merely comparing people who have experience with meditation to those who don't. A handful of studies have tackled this issue head on by employing controlled longitudinal designs. In these studies, researchers track participants over time as they learn to meditate. The findings suggest that meditating for just a few weeks, or even days, changes the structure and activity of the brain [7]. Most of these longitudinal studies compare meditation training to a control condition involving a waitlist or practice of a tangential skill such as reading or progressive relaxation. Such controlled designs strengthen the claim that the observed brain changes came about specifically from meditation training. Furthermore, some of the regions that have been shown to change following meditation training overlap with the changes observed in meditation experts, lending further support to the idea that these brain areas may play a role in meditation. Stimulating some of these brain areas in mice has even been shown to make these mice exhibit less apparently anxious behavior—leading to the first so-called "rodent model" of meditation (though the model would be better described as a meditation model of rodent behavior) [8].

Nonetheless, these findings should be taken with a grain of salt. Crucially, most of the neuroimaging studies on meditation have very small sample sizes. Neuroimaging studies with fewer than 20 participants per group—which includes the vast majority of studies on meditation—have very low statistical power to accurately detect all but the largest of effects in a limited set of brain regions [9]. Low statistical power not only increases the chances of missing real effects (type II error), but also substantially inflates the risk of finding spurious results that nonetheless pass statistical threshold (type I error)—see Chapter 12 for more detail on this topic. Findings from small samples should really be treated as preliminary until they are replicated in independent groups with more statistical power. Yet, few of the longitudinal findings on brain changes in meditation have been replicated. Compound this situation with the trendiness of meditation science and the fact that negative findings often go unpublished, and you have the perfect recipe for a field at high risk of false positives [10].

One way to partially mitigate these concerns is through meta-analysis, an approach that amalgamates all of the available data in a scientific field to see if reliable patterns emerge. A few recent meta-analyses have suggested that there may be some consistent brain changes across neuroimaging studies of meditation [6,11]. However, the software that was used to conduct these meta-analyses had a bug that accidentally inflated statistical effects [12]. Unfortunately the meta-analyses were published before this bug was discovered and fixed, so there is good reason to think that the results may be overstated. This is a poignant illustration of the complex statistical and interpretive issues that permeate a young scientific field such as neuroimaging [13]. Given the tenuous nature of the neuroscientific evidence concerning meditation, it seems misguided to think that the reported brain changes are more meaningful than other observable effects, such as changes in behavior, subjective experience, or clinical symptoms.

The mindful brain in social and bodily context

Even if we assume that the brain changes reported in neuroimaging studies of meditation are robust, there remains a deeper conceptual problem with the idea that we can map (let alone reduce) complex behaviors or mental processes to changes in particular regions or networks of the brain [14]). There is more to mindfulness than just adopting a brain state or training a brain pattern. Mindfulness is not an internal cognitive process that maps neatly onto the brain; it's a complex orchestration of cognitive skills embodied in a particular social context [5,15].

Consider parenting as an analogy. Parenting skills certainly depend on the brain—and practicing them changes the brain—but they are not private mental processes and do not exist inside the brain. Specific patterns of brain activity might correlate with being a good parent in a given context, but these brain

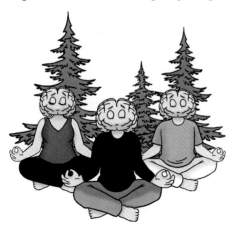

patterns alone hardly explain what it is to be a good parent. Good parenting isn't inside the brain; it's a way in which the whole person (including the brain) is engaged in the world. Moreover, what counts as good parenting differs depending on the culture. So appealing to the brain simply won't tell us what it means to be a good parent. To bring this into view we need a wider perspective, one that takes into consideration the context of the whole person as well as the social and cultural environment. The same is true for mindfulness.

Social context shapes mindfulness meditation in many ways: it influences what people hope to achieve from meditating, how they arrange their environment and body when they practice, and who else is around when they meditate—to name but a few examples. All of these social factors likely impact meditation experience in a multitude of ways that scientists are only just beginning to understand [15,16]. For example, one recent study examined how expectations influence the outcomes of a simple mindful breath awareness exercise [17]. Before the mindfulness exercise the researchers told half of the participants (all of whom were new to meditation) that the practice would immediately improve their attention skills. The other participants were told instead that the meditation would exhaust the brain's limited attention capacity. Only participants who were led to expect positive changes showed improvements in attention (in fact, negative expectations actually impaired attention performance). This finding highlights the importance of social beliefs and expectations in shaping the outcomes of mindfulness practice [18]. It's not just the instructions we follow that determine our experience of meditation. It's also the expectations and beliefs we glean from our social context. The "meaning" we ascribe to practices, including mindfulness meditation, seems to play a key role in shaping our thinking, our healing, and even our biology [19].

The body also plays a crucial role in mindfulness meditation [20.21]. Many traditions of meditative practice consider the posture of the body to act as a mirror of the mind [22]. When attention dulls, the posture slackens. When thinking becomes agitated or aggressive, the muscles become stiff and taut. Mind and body are bound together. Modern neuroscientific studies support this key insight of ancient meditative traditions. Recent findings demonstrate that bodily posture (e.g., sitting upright versus lying down) profoundly alters baseline brain activity [23]. Moreover, some of the brain regions that are most susceptible to posture-dependent changes are the same regions that are often linked to meditation (such as regions of the "default-mode network"). The very act of lying down for an fMRI scan, or sitting down to meditate, changes how the brain operates (see Chapter 10). How then can we hope to understand the meditating brain without appreciating the meditating body?

Conclusion

The popularity of the *mindful brain* says a great deal about our culture's fascination with scientific evidence and about our eagerness to reduce the richness of subjective experience to a physical substrate that we can see and measure. The allure of neuroimaging feeds into this neurocentric view of mindfulness, which in turn reinforces our internally focused approach to well-being. But mental wellness depends on more than what's inside our heads. Moving past a neurocentric view of mindfulness promises not only to improve the science of meditation, but also to counteract the pernicious idea that taking care of our minds is just a matter of regulating our own internal states. Part of what meditative practice reveals is that our minds are intrinsically tied up with our bodies and with the larger social and ecological contexts in which we are embedded. We hope for a science of mindfulness that would make us more, not less, mindful of how our brains fit into this bigger picture.

Additional readings

A journal issue dedicated to thinking about how cultural context shapes the experiences and outcomes of meditative practices: Kirmayer LJ. Mindfulness in cultural context. Transcult Psychiatry 2015;52(4):447−69.

A scientific review arguing for the importance of the body in meditation: Khoury B, Knäuper B, Pagnini F, Trent N, Chiesa A, Carrière K. Embodied mindfulness. Mindfulness 2017;8(5):1160−71.

A historian addressing the importance of cultural context as a mechanism in meditation: McMahan DL. Meditation, Buddhism, and science. How meditation works: theorizing the role of cultural context in Buddhist contemplative practices. New York: Oxford University Press; 2017. p. 21−46. Chapter 3.

An in-depth exploration of the central ideas in this chapter: Thompson E. Meditation, Buddhism, and science. Looping effects and the cognitive science of mindfulness meditation. New York: Oxford University Press; 2017. p. 47−61. Chapter 4.

"Backed by neuroscience": How brain imaging sells

22

Lauren Dahl and Amir Raz

If someone showed you a scan of your brain, would you be able to interpret it? Could you locate the subcortical areas involved in motor control or your anterior cingulate cortex? Would you know how to identify subtle signs of damage, atrophy, or neurodegeneration? The average person rarely knows this stuff. That's why we rely on brain researchers and health care professionals to help us understand what's going on. However, sometimes these experts abuse their expertise: some overestimate the power of neuroimaging and our current knowledge of the brain, others advertise treatments and products based on questionable technology and ambiguous research.

Neuroimaging provides visual depictions of the brain based on a range of different technologies such as magnetic resonance imaging (MRI) and positron emission tomography. This process has led to countless advances in medicine and research. We tend to put more trust in products and services "backed by neuroscience" or "supported by brain imaging research" because they seem to carry a stamp of scientific approval. But these claims occasionally gloss over the very real limitations of current technologies and scientific knowledge.

Historically, phrenology offered a popular model of the brain with distinct anatomical locations for functions such as conscientiousness and self-esteem; later, Freudian psychoanalysis represented the leading way of viewing the mind as well as relationships with the self and others. Today, cognitive brain researchers and behavioral scientists have firmly dismissed phrenology and regard many a psychoanalysis idea as outdated. Brain imaging has provided a largely objective way to test hypotheses by conducting empirical research. In doing so, we have moved past many pseudoscientific practices and ideas. Nevertheless, a few practitioners still manage to use brain imaging injudiciously.

One clinician who holds bona fide medical credentials, for example, founded a network of commercial clinics promoting neuroimaging as the gold standard of diagnostics. Using single positron emission computed tomography—an early imaging technique which involves injecting participants with a radioactive dye and then using computer software to render glossy brain graphics that colorfully illustrate blood flow—this physician claims to diagnose and distinguish between several different types of attention disorders, different types of anxiety and depression, as well as weight issues,

Casting Light on the Dark Side of Brain Imaging. DOI: https://doi.org/10.1016/B978-0-12-816179-1.00022-0

addiction, marital conflict, and a wide-range of other conditions [1]. Running at least six clinics and having published a number of bestselling books, this practitioner often speaks at live events and on television, sometimes under the label "America's most popular psychiatrist." One of the infomercials for (and by) his clinic aired nearly 1300 times on the public broadcasting service (PBS) stations across the United States, reaching more than 75% of television households [2]. And yet, major clinical societies and research centers, including the American Psychiatric Association, debunk these advertised claims, and experts from the National Institutes of Mental Health, the American College of Radiology, and various other academic institutions have explicitly spoken out against this practice [1]. It seems that for many people, a few published books, TV appearances, and a nice smile hold more weight than widespread expert opinion based on libraries-worth of scientific evidence.

The emerging field of Critical Neuroscience [3] cautions against overestimating the power of imaging tools and serves as a knee-jerk reaction to demonstrations showing that even a dead fish can elicit activity on fMRI scans [4]. After all, imag-

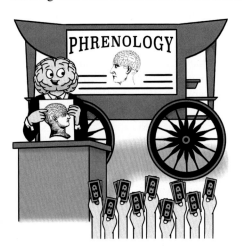

ing methods are limited by signal-to-noise ratios and other imprecisions: they cannot always provide a perfectly detailed picture of the brain. Moreover, even if researchers had a pristine image of the brain, they wouldn't be able to explain and interpret every single aspect of it, simply because we still have major lacunae in our knowledge. Thus conclusions drawn from neuroimaging assays have the potential to overpromise and underdeliver, and we can't always be sure that advertising based on "neuroscience" presents a full story. Advertisements may truthfully state that products are the subject of a study or based on scientific research, without clarifying what the research shows or how closely the studies relate to the product. Coupled with handpicked testimonials, such marketing strategies can effectively lead consumers to make inaccurate inferences, to the benefit of the company. Thus we must always balance two concerning trends: the overpowering influence of brain-related technology on our ability to make decisions [5] and the possible dangers of being an uninformed consumer [6].

For another example, consider the story of Lumosity (Lumos Labs Inc., 2017), which represents one of the more visible brain training companies in North America. For about US$15 per month, or a lifetime membership of US$300, Lumosity grants you access to an expanding variety of games through its web application: matching games aiming to engage memory and processing speed, visual searches targeting attention, and games demanding timed mental calculation. From Internet ads to television and radio commercials, the company successfully leveraged a forceful marketing campaign suggesting that their games can help delay the onset of Alzheimer's and other forms of age-related decline [7]. With people living longer and becoming more aware of the perils of aging, Lumosity's campaign appeared to offer a solution to their customers' desires to stave off cognitive impairment.

The case of Lumosity speaks to the effectiveness of deceptive advertising, although research findings from experiments on brain training challenge many of these marketing claims. In early 2016 Lumosity agreed to a $2 million settlement with the Federal Trade Commission for "charges alleging that they deceived consumers with unfounded claims that [their] games can help users perform better at work and in school, and reduce or delay cognitive impairment associated with age and other serious health conditions" [7] This legal process signaled a low point, at least in scientific merit, for one of the most aggressively marketed commercial brain training programs to date.

In 2015 less than a year before the Lumosity settlement, the Canadian Broadcasting Corporation (CBC) approached neuroscientist Adrian Owen to examine Lumosity as part of an investigation on "mind games" [8] (CBC, 2015), to help determine whether there was truth in their advertising. Owen, who has previously engaged in a similar production with the British Broadcasting Corporation [9], publicly broadcasted the message that computerized brain training games have yet to show real generalizable benefits to, for example, inhibitory control, emotional regulation, and resilience. Although neither the CBC nor the BBC program represents a rigorous scientific experiment, the sentiment remains relevant and has been reverberating more formally in peer-reviewed publications [10].

Cognitive training and imaging of the living human brain (as opposed to the liver, spleen, or heart) appeal to most people because these methods seem to provide an intuitive glimpse into our human inner core. Unfortunately, some current applications of neuroscience have many limitations. And yet, at least a few doctors and companies seem to take advantage of these gaps. As people live longer lives, the worry concerning aging and the associated physical and mental changes tend to increase. We should be both hopeful and skeptical of what fields such as brain training and neuroimaging can offer. We must let the evidence, not infomercials, guide us.

Additional readings

An exposé on the notorious SPECT clinics: Bernstein R. Head case: why has P.B.S. Promoted controversial shrink Dr. Daniel Amen? Observer; 2016.

An analysis of recent advancements in the field of critical neuroscience: Choudhury S, Slaby J. Critical neuroscience: a handbook of the social and cultural contexts of neuroscience; 2011.

An article on the limitations of fMRI: Ozdemir M. Controversial science of brain imaging. Sci. Am. 2012.

Section VI

What next?

From regions to networks: Neuroimaging approaches to mapping brain organization

Ricky Burns, Daniel S. Margulies and Philipp Haueis

When most people think of neuroimaging an iconic image comes immediately to mind: a gray brain overlaid with a brightly colored blob. To create these brain maps, neuroscientists record activity from a living human brain using tools such as functional magnetic resonance imaging (fMRI) and positron emission tomography (PET). Without a conceptual framework to interpret the activity recorded by these techniques, however, neuroimaging maps would remain meaningless. Cognitive psychology, which studies mental processes using tasks that probe our abilities to perceive, attend, and remember, provides this framework. With the help of cognitive tasks, neuroscientists have mapped specialized functions in the brain over the last four decades. In this chapter, we highlight the limits of this task-based approach and explain why researchers now complement it with a novel, network-based approach to understand brain organization. Counterintuitively, this novel approach relies on studying brain activity in the absence of task demands, an approach therefore referred to as "resting-state" fMRI.

The task-based approach assumes that cognitive functions correspond to specific brain regions. But with recent innovations that allow peoples' brain activity to be analyzed while they simply relax, researchers have started to study the brain's organizational architecture independent of these cognitive assumptions. Neuroscientists view such resting-state studies as part of a larger approach called "connectomics" because it emphasizes the structural, functional, and topological properties of connections between brain regions [1,2]. Although a relatively new method, many researchers believe that connectomics provides the field of brain mapping with an alternative framework based in network science and neuroanatomy. The emerging field of connectomics offers the possibility to replace or at least complement the prior foundation of brain mapping in cognitive psychology [3,4].

Modern neuroimaging is the most recent advance in a long line of methods for mapping brain organization. Before the popularization of brain images began

Casting Light on the Dark Side of Brain Imaging. DOI: https://doi.org/10.1016/B978-0-12-816179-1.00023-2

in the 1970s, there was a 100-year history of mapping brain organization by chemically staining dead brain tissue, recording brainwaves with electrophysiology equipment, and artificially stimulating the brain with surgically implanted electrodes. The primary advantage of these more invasive methods is that they can bring microscopic properties of the brain to light and provide gold-standard methods for precisely mapping brain activity. In contrast, PET and MRI can only reveal a general area of activation, which typically contains millions of neurons [5].

With that said, the advantage of neuroimaging lies in its capacity to study complex cognitive functions that cannot be inferred from animal models. Because it is unethical to implant electrodes into healthy volunteers or remove parts of their brain, we often rely on less invasive methods when studying human brain function. Early cognitive neuroscience studies used cognitive tasks to study higher-level human functions such as reading, working memory, and attention. These studies aimed to map functional modules in the brain using task-related activity. Such mappings have enabled researchers to propose models and mechanisms for how localized brain activity contributes to complex cognition processes and patterns of behavior. However, in so doing, researchers focused solely on the activity induced by tasks and discarded ongoing fluctuations in brain activity, which were considered to be nothing more than noise.

Researchers investigating this "noise" in the fMRI signal were surprised to discover that it was in fact highly organized [6]. This discovery led to the concept of "resting state networks"—brain systems that are synchronized in their ongoing spontaneous activity, even in the absence of any specific task demands. Resting-state fMRI thus enabled the investigation of brain function outside the conceptual framework of cognitive psychology, as now researchers could probe network organization without relying on specific functional states. Although critics initially resisted the idea of studying brain function at rest, numerous studies have since demonstrated its utility and validity for characterizing large-scale functional systems [7—10].

One critical finding from this line of research is that cognitive functions do not map in a clear one-to-one correspondence with resting state networks. It was this finding that made researchers reexamine the conceptual foundations of brain mapping. Why should we assume that the brain necessarily aligns with the modules of cognitive psychology [11]? This assumption has not held true when analyzing the multiple network interactions that take place during higher-level cognitive functions such as memory retrieval, mind wandering, or even reading. These results suggest that modern cognitive psychology may use categories that do not divide the brain into biologically meaningful parts. It is for this reason that current neuroscience research is making a dramatic shift toward methods that focus on brain connectivity. The most appealing tools to date have come from combining network science with large datasets of functional and structural connectivity data.

Network analyses reduce a system's complexity to a map of its connections. In neuroscience, we use graph theory to describe the brain as a network of interconnected cells, circuits, or areas. Neuroscientists refer to this mapping of neural connections at different scales "connectomics" [1]. Connectomics researchers often use structural and functional MRI to visualize the brain's organization as a series of large-scale

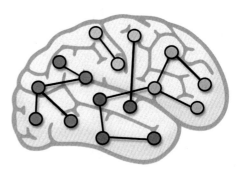

networks. This approach does not presuppose simple correspondence between cognitive capacities and specific areas of the brain, but rather lets the brain tell us how it is organized. In this way, connectomics provides a contrasting conceptual framework from the assumptions of cognitive psychology.

The shift toward using connectivity as a basis for brain mapping has fostered new ambitions based largely on these methods. Notably the Human Connectome Project [12], a 5-year $40 million U.S. National Institute of Health grant, recently resulted in a publication in a leading research journal, *Nature* of a novel brain map [13]. A continued commitment to this development in methodology along with a returned interest in cortical anatomy has also enabled neuroimaging researchers to characterize the layout of fiber pathways in the living human brain. With advances in existing technologies and increased collaborations between large study groups, the field of neuroimaging is finding success in deciphering brain organization through a connectivity approach.

While these advances are reasons to celebrate, we should acknowledge that conceptualizing the brain through the network approach remains one strategy among many others. Just as any method has its drawbacks, the network method has potential to introduce bias due to the difficulty in controlling the resting-state environment. Currently an area of concern going forward is that there is no optimal method to control what a participant is thinking about in an MRI scanner. Some people might drift off and daydream about lunch, others might focus on the stress of entering a brain scanner. Different mental states no doubt impact the activity patterns of a resting-state fMRI scan. With that said, while the task-based approach requires individuals to focus on a task for a short while, this method does not ensure that the participant is exclusively focused on the task at hand. Suppose your task is to push a button every time you see the number "3" on a screen when laying in the scanner. Because it is hardly cognitively demanding, most participants may start thinking about other things while executing the task more or less automatically. So while both approaches require better control of experimental conditions, the crucial difference between the methods is that the task-based approach is largely hypothesis driven, while the connectomic approach is largely exploratory and data-driven [14].

While the task-based approach requires a cognitive hypothesis that predicts which changes in brain activity are induced by the task, the connectomic approach does not decide beforehand which data patterns from the testing phase are relevant.

The exploratory connectomic approach can therefore contribute to the formation of novel concepts to describe brain organization as a complement to the concepts of cognitive psychology [11]. Besides continued improvement of the two approaches most discussed in this chapter, there must also be a continued dedication to the development of other autonomous methods such as high-resolution structural methods—a modern equivalent of the histology (chemical staining) techniques that proved so fruitful for mapping brain organization in the last century. A recent example is the use of high-resolution MRI signals as markers for microanatomical features like myelin, the tissue that insulates neurons.

Just as any scientific model requires adapting to newly acquired information, the models of the brain must do the same. Modern cognitive psychology has brought neuroscience to where it is now, and it remains crucial in shaping ongoing neuroscience research. To complement concepts drawn from cognitive psychology, researchers are beginning to develop concepts about brain organization based on categories and mechanisms derived from the brain itself [4]. This could reshape how we see the brain in the future: not only as an information processing device, but also as a physiological apparatus that maintains and repairs itself along with the rest of the body [15]. Currently, network science possesses some of the most promising tools to achieve this goal, and its recent results suggest that the field is progressing toward greater discoveries.

Although we mainly contrasted task-based and connectomic approaches with each other, we emphasize that ultimately, neuroscience will only progress by integrating both network and cognitive psychological concepts. Indeed, studies that compared resting state fMRI patterns with cognitive activation maps show that there is a systematic relation between spontaneous network and local task-evoked activity in the brain [9]. Examples such as these show that no one set of concepts or methods is sufficient to fully understand the morphological, chemical, physiological, cognitive, computational, and network properties of the brain. By expanding the perspective of neuroimaging beyond classical cognitive psychology, connectomics is but one step toward a truly multidisciplinary understanding of how the brain works.

Additional readings

A broad overview of connectomic methods from one of the pioneers of network neuroscience:
    Sporns O: Discovering the connectome. Cambridge, MA: MIT Press; 2012.
A landmark paper of the Human Connectome Project, which describes a novel brain map created using multiple large-scale datasets, including resting-state fMRI: Glasser MF, Coalson TS, Robinson EC, et al. A multi-modal parcellation of human cerebral cortex. Nature 2016;536(7615):171−8.

Whole-brain modeling of neuroimaging data: Moving beyond correlation to causation

24

Morten L. Kringelbach and Gustavo Deco

Neuroimaging has offered an unprecedented window on human brain activity. While this advance has led to great expectations, many neuroscientists have grown increasingly frustrated with the lack of causal insights that this technique has provided into human brain function, in turn, leading to heated discussions on the potential rise of neophrenology [1–4]. Elsewhere in this book, you can read about the apparent failure of brain imaging to tell us much new or meaningful about thinking and cognition in general. Such views are true to a certain extent; brain imaging often takes indirect measures of neural activity such as blood flow and, just because such brain measures correlate with behavioral output, does not mean that they cause the output. But, these new tools *do* measure important information about brain activity that could potentially tell us a great deal about brain and mind.

In physics, scientists have long argued that in order for science to progress, we need to ask the right question, collect the right data, and then build a model that explains the data. Without an adequate model, we are merely observers lacking the necessary deep understanding of the laws governing how the data is generated. Current brain imaging experiments tend to collect data and establish correlations rather than develop models and uncover fundamental principles and causal mechanisms of brain function. In order to use human brain imaging to discover causal triggers and key pathways involved in brain diseases, we will need to move beyond the current state of correlative neuroimaging and start creating causal models. For conditions where animal models are less than optimal—such as neuropsychiatric disorders—we can create and test new theoretical computational models of brain function to make sense of the human brain and attempt to repair it.

These computer models of the living human brain can be used in a similar manner to animal models—to predict the causal contribution of different brain regions to behavior. Computational models can also provide deeper insights into what is

Casting Light on the Dark Side of Brain Imaging. DOI: https://doi.org/10.1016/B978-0-12-816179-1.00024-4

being computed when we attempt to navigate our complex physical and social environments. They hold potential where animal models have had little success. For example, for complex human neuropsychiatric disorders where animal models alone are insufficient for gaining new insights into underlying mechanisms and potential treatments. Such efforts could instead benefit from causal modeling of human brain imaging data [5].

Modeling the causal dynamics of brain states

Just as meteorologists input data concerning humidity, temperature, and wind patterns into computational models to predict future weather, neuroscientists can use whole-brain computational models to predict output in terms of brain activity and behavior. In both cases, the models are based on decades of research and are updated as new data comes in. The development of new whole-brain computational models has drawn inspiration not only from theoretical physics, but also from the much earlier ideas of the medieval philosopher Thomas Aquinas who, in the spirit of Aristotle, wrote "Quidquid recipitur ad modum recipientis recipitur," which roughly translates into the idea that the container (or recipient) shapes the content.

The Aristotelian idea that containers shape content can be directly linked to how spontaneous brain activity is tied to the underlying structure of the *connectome*, which describes the anatomical connections in the white-matter fibers linking neurons together [6−11] (see chapter 23). The energy landscape made possible by the connectome is often called the spontaneous or resting-state activity of the brain [12,13] and can be thought of as the ongoing dynamics of connected networks that underlie brain function.

A series of state-of-the-art studies computationally modeled the resting-state brain using three main ingredients: (1) a parcellation of the human brain into a set number of regions, (2) the anatomical connectivity between these regions, and (3) the neural dynamics in each region [5,9,10,14−18]. When creating a model, researchers need to make important choices for each of these ingredients. For example, how many regions should we parcel the brain into best estimate its topographic organization [4]? How should we best estimate the anatomical connectivity from imperfect measurements like diffusion functional magnetic resonance imaging (fMRI) [19]? Should the model capture the average neural activity across a region or the dynamic fluctuations throughout time [10]? Once these choices have been taken, the model is simply fitted to the experimental data by changing only *one* global scaling parameter, which scales the underlying anatomical connectivity estimated from the empirical data. If this global scaling parameter is very small, the model will use very weak overall connectivity and can only generate weak dynamics, which will not fit the empirical data—except perhaps if the data are from a comatose patient. On the other hand, if the global scaling parameter is very large so that the global connectivity is also large, the model would better fit the data of an epileptic seizure brain than that of a normal person. Still, at the optimal point of the global scaling parameter, the model has been shown to capture the dynamics of resting-state data in normal people with a remarkable accuracy of around 80%—depending, of course, on the quality of choices made for the model.

Understanding the physics of complex systems is helpful for better characterizing the performance of these models. The concept of *metastability* is crucial when discussing the optimal state of the energy landscape of the brain. Metastability is a measure of how variable brain states are as a function of time. In other words, how the synchronization in activity between the different brain regions fluctuates across time. Research has demonstrated that the normal brain operates at optimal 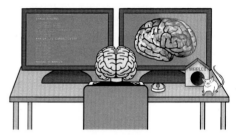 metastability and properly executes time-critical neural computations that allow animals to survive [9,20,21]. The complex brain activity that occurs during rest and cognition plays out on the background of the brain's structural connectivity. Crucially the brain has to balance the exploration and exploitation of this dynamical landscape of possibilities to ensure stability in the long term. This is achieved though balancing integration and segregation processing in order to function optimally [15].

Fitting a whole-brain model to neuroimaging data opens vast potential in terms of revealing the underlying causal mechanisms that give rise to the energy landscape of the brain [10,22]. Researchers can systematically perturb or "lesion" the computer model to test which regions and networks are essential for generating certain dynamics. As an example, we can quantify the level of binding of information in the human brain by ranking regions according to their level of temporal integration. We showed that lesioning elements of the whole-brain model can be used to demonstrate a causal relationship between the contribution of the binding regions to ensuing brain activity [23]. Neuroimaging research on the diseased brain shows that the energy landscape has become unbalanced [24]. Using whole-brain models to discover the changes underlying the unbalance can help in finding the best ways to rebalance the brain [25].

Patients with Parkinson's disease provide a tangible example of where whole-brain modeling has been useful. Deep brain stimulation of the subthalamic nucleus can help alleviate the symptoms of these patients. While careful research in animal models made this important intervention possible, it still wasn't clear why stimulating this brain target is so effective at alleviating symptoms and whether better ways to rebalance the Parkinsonian brain exist. With the arrival of a few important technical advances, scientists can now record brain imaging data from Parkinsonian patients while their deep brain stimulators are turned on or off [26]. Subsequently, we used whole-brain computations to model the energy landscape of brain activity when the stimulator is on and off [27]. This experiment enabled us to find the causal networks that change with stimulation of the subthalamic nucleus. Using this careful computer modeling, we can also identify new candidate brain regions that may lead to even better outcomes when stimulated.

While such whole-brain computational models may not currently tell us much about thinking or cognition in the healthy or diseased brain, it is also not clear that cognition is all that important for rebalancing the diseased brain. Instead, it may suffice to use whole-brain models to find new ways to recreate the normal brain's energy landscape that is necessary for rebalancing the brain, which in turn will help cognition and alleviate suffering. Take the example of neuropsychiatric disorders where, unlike Parkinson's disease, we do not currently have a good understanding of why the brain has become unbalanced but where whole-brain modeling may offer novel targets. Yet, we should note that the rebalancing of the brain need not require invasive deep brain electrodes; but could also come through drugs, cognitive behavioral therapy, or even psychotherapy [28]. There is important scope for using whole-brain modeling to track the changes in the energy landscape as a patient improves after an intervention, and further, to causally identify the key nodes and networks involved in this change. We have recently added a fourth ingredient to the models: neurotransmitters which serve to dynamically change the brain's energy landscape [29]. These models could open long-term exciting possibilities for rational drug discovery and design intended for neuropsychiatric disorders.

Conclusion

In order to fulfill the great expectations many people have of human brain imaging, over the last decade we have worked on developing a novel framework based on increasingly sophisticated whole-brain models [6–9]. These models have allowed us to gain a much better mechanistic understanding of human brain function [15]. We have created powerful computer models in silico and accurately reproduced human brain activity as measured with a combination of many different neuroimaging techniques. Researchers can now treat these computational models like animal models, and systematic lesion and stimulate them to accurately describe many of the mechanisms underlying human brain activity [10].

Overall, combining careful experimental brain imaging methods with state-of-the-art causal whole-brain modeling can perhaps, for the first time, reveal the mechanisms responsible for any form of brain processing in health and disease. This advance opens the possibility for new treatments and perhaps even eudaimonia and better lives—especially if coupled with early interventions.

Additional readings

Deep brain stimulation is a powerful tool for rebalancing the brain as you can read more about in: Kringelbach ML, Aziz TZ. Sparking recovery with brain "pacemakers". Sci Am Mind 2008;6:36−43.

Whole-brain models can offer new insights into neuropsychiatric disorders: Deco G, Kringelbach ML. Great expectations: using whole-brain computational connectomics for understanding neuropsychiatric disorders. Neuron 2014;84:892−905.

You can play around with whole-brain modelling yourself using the virtual brain: <https://www.thevirtualbrain.org>.

This book argues that emotion and not cognition is what matters when it comes to good life; and thus what is important is to find ways to rebalance these emotional networks: Kringelbach ML, Phillips H. Emotion. Pleasure and pain in the brain. Oxford: Oxford University Press; 2014.

Connecting networks to neurons

25

Michael I. Posner

Pictures of the human brain have been enormously helpful. Just as the image of earth from space helped give rise to earth day, colorful images of the living human brain influenced the congressional declaration of *"The Decade of the Brain,"* made in the United States in the 1990s. Brain images, such as those depicted in Fig. 25.1, result from the activity of many thousands of nerve cells working together. A dream of neuroscience is to bridge the gap from these large-scale activation maps to the work of groups of cells and even to single neurons and axons such as those depicted in Fig. 25.2. This chapter discusses research on attention networks that might help connect neuroimaging to cellular and molecular events.

Since the early days of neuroimaging, I have been most involved in studying attentional networks. Experiments from various fields, including behavioral, devel-

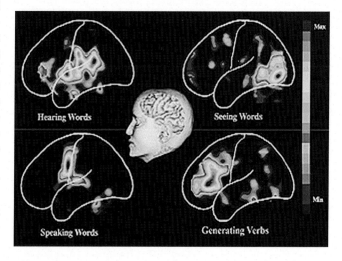

Figure 25.1 Neuroimages in bright colors of brain areas active during various language tasks. Contributed by Michael Posner.

opmental, and imaging research, have converged to establish three brain networks involved in attention. These networks achieve an alert state (alerting), orient to sensory events (orienting), and control conflict between competing response tendencies (executive) [1]. Each of these networks involves mostly separate brain areas although the networks frequently work in concert when individuals perform a task.

Perhaps most remarkable in these efforts is that merely asking someone to exercise control over their thoughts or feelings activates attentional networks. By now, many studies have established this by asking individuals to attend to visual stimuli rather than simultaneous auditory events [2], to create a visual image [3], to avoid

Casting Light on the Dark Side of Brain Imaging. DOI: https://doi.org/10.1016/B978-0-12-816179-1.00025-6

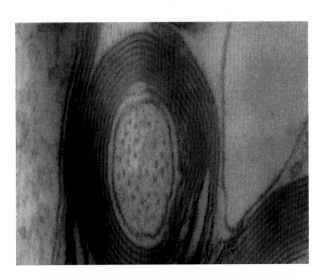

Figure 25.2 A picture of an individual connective fiber (axon) with the surrounding myelin rings as insulation. Electron micrograph 16K magnification. Contributed by Dr. Denise Piscopo.

negative [4] or positive reactions [5] to a stimulus, or even to control the order of mental operations when performing a task [6]. In these studies a complex attentional network is activated (including the anterior cingulate, anterior insula, and striatum), in addition to the specific sensory or motor areas of the brain which are directly involved in the specific task. Since these areas are activated in experiments involving instructions to control, it seems reasonable to conclude that they are also used in the implementation of our natural wishes and desires in addition to responding to the instructions of the researcher.

Not only do attentional brain networks correlate with specific tasks, they are also important for our success in life. Tasks which activate these brain areas are related to ratings, both by oneself and others, on how well someone can control their thoughts and feelings in daily life [7]. From such ratings in young children, studies have successfully predicted their later success in income, health, and social relations as adults [8]. The skills and brain networks involved in self-control, moreover, are far from fixed; they can be taught, for example, through computerized tasks and mindfulness meditation.

In studies on humans, using diffusion tensor imaging, mindfulness meditation as well as other purely cognitive tasks has altered the connectivity of attention networks by improving the ability of axons to connect neurons. How could the purely mental activity of meditation, which involves keeping your attention fixed in the present and not allowing it to wander, result in a physical change in the white matter that surrounds axons? Several studies recording from scalp electrodes (EEG) have shown that meditation training increases rhythmic oscillations (4−8 Hz, theta range) over mid line frontal brain areas involved in attentional control. This finding led to the hypothesis [9] that theta stimulation activated dormant nonneuronal brain cells (oligodendrocytes) that lead to increases in myelin that surrounds axons.

To test this hypothesis, we can use a technique called optogenetics. This method uses lasers to activate or suppress cells that have been rendered sensitive to light [10]. Currently, optogenetics can only be done in animal models, but it is possible that less invasive versions may be available in the future.

Optogenetics and animal models may not be overly useful for studying language tasks like those shown in Fig. 25.1, but we can use them to study many interesting human tasks like those involving attention networks of alerting, orienting, and conflict resolution. For example, we can directly stimulate or inhibit neurons in the anterior cingulate of mice and observe how this procedure alters the kind of attentional control found in studies of human self-regulation (for an example, see [11]). After controlling the output and frequency of firing from the anterior cingulate with optogenetics, we have used electromicrographs to observe the change in white matter, as shown in Fig. 25.2. By relating the human and mouse studies, we can move beyond the idea of self-regulation as a purely psychological level of explanation and toward a detailed account of how neurons influence the brain networks that lead to self-control.

Control networks in the brain seem to be active even when participants are at rest and not carrying out any task [12] (see chapter 23). Researchers have imaged these large-scale brain networks of attention to trace their development from infancy to old age. To get a more detailed understanding of these networks, scientists have imaged individual brain cells in rodents and shown the role of slow oscillatory brain rhythms in supporting the activity of large-scale networks [13]. These advancements give promise of a molecular understanding of how seemingly spontaneous activity of brain networks at rest can organize during brain development.

Being able to see images of brain networks provides a strong visual experience which is perhaps often more persuasive than it should be. To increase the insights we can gain from these images, researchers can use brain stimulation, animal models, and computational models (see chapter 24)—to investigate different levels of analyses. Linking large-scale human networks to the underlying cellular structure will not answer all the interesting questions of the human brain; it is, however, a critical next step in our effort to further such understanding.

Additional readings

Raichle ME. A paradigm shift in functional brain imaging. J Neurosci 2009;29/41:12729–34.
Rothbart MK. Becoming who we are. New York: Guilford; 2011.
Posner MI. Attention in a social world. New York: Oxford Univ. Press; 2012.

High field magnetic resonance imaging

26

Alayar Kangarlu

On July 3, 1977, magnetic resonance imaging (MRI) was first used to acquire images of a living human [1]. Since then, MRI has consistently provided noninvasive images of the human body and helped clinicians and scientists diagnose various pathologies and study their physiology. Contrary to the early expectations of the medical community, however, MRI did not quickly evolve into a tool for independent diagnosis of diseases and disorders. One culprit was the inherently low sensitivity caused by the low magnetic field strength of these scanners which stood at 1.5 T (Tesla) for two decades. With the debut of a scanner operating at 8 T in 1998, high field (HF) MRI became a reality. Today, most hospitals have 3 T clinical scanners and the standard of HF research has become 7 T scanners. HF scanners, which range anywhere from 7 to 11.7 T, have shown the potential to examine the functional anatomy of the brain; for example, to determine parts of the brain that do functions such as thought, speech, movement, and sensation; to study the consequences of trauma, stroke, or degenerative disease on brain function; to monitor the growth of brain tumors; and to help plan radiation therapy, surgery, or other invasive treatments on the brain. To expand these capabilities, the science, engineering, and safety of these new scanners are critical issues which must be developed in parallel. In particular the role of radio frequency (RF) coils, magnetic susceptibility, and pulse sequences is prominent in this regard. In addition, HF MRI has the potential to go beyond imaging of brain and develop sensitivity for direct physiological processes, and ultimately become a

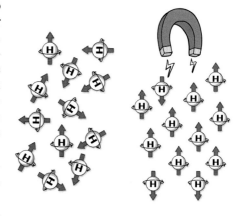

tool for cellular and molecular imaging. In this context, HF MRI could provide new insight into the etiology and pathophysiology of many diseases and also help expand our understanding of basic biology.

Casting Light on the Dark Side of Brain Imaging. DOI: https://doi.org/10.1016/B978-0-12-816179-1.00026-8

History

MRI is a unique imaging technique that produces its signal by inducing a magnetic field that alters atomic properties (the spin state of the protons within atomic nuclei [2,3]). Hydrogen is the most abundant element in the human body and has ideal magnetic properties that allow us to produce MRI images. The resolution of MRI images depends on the smallest volume from which we can obtain a signal that is stronger than noise; this comparison is known as the signal-to-noise ratio (SNR) [4]. Since 1977 when MRI scanners were introduced into clinical settings and bio-medical research, the minimum SNR necessary to produce diagnostically viable images has set the strength of the magnets used in these scanners at 1.5 T. Compromise on this field strength was due to engineering issues in manufacturing stronger magnets, the troubling effects of high magnetic fields on image quality, and the difficulty in constructing of high quality RF coils. In 1998 the news of an upcoming 8 T human MRI scanner at Ohio State University (OSU) took the medical imaging community by storm [5]. Besides the issues surrounding engineering and image quality, at that time, safety appeared to be an insurmountable obstacle for any human exposed to such high-strength magnetic fields [6,7]. The OSU group conducted a series of seminal work on MRI safety that convinced the scientific community and governmental regulatory bodies that there was no significant risk associated with scanning human subjects in a HF MRI [8]. This research was a major step in bringing all the advantages of HF beyond high-resolution anatomical MRI and to other modalities that use the same MRI scanners, such as fMRI [9], spectroscopy [10], and diffusion tensor imaging [11].

Imaging brain function

Since the early 1990s, functional magnetic resonance imaging (fMRI) has become a powerful tool in neuroscience research. Presently, there are hundreds of 3 T scanners used for research in the world. They are primarily used to measure the function of the brain (via fMRI studies) rather than investigation of anatomy alone (via MRI). In addition, there are about 50 HF scanners operating at field strengths of 7 T and higher. These HF scanners are technically capable of shedding light on the neuronal activity of the brain via the blood oxygen level dependent (BOLD) contrast which is a hemodynamic response to neuronal activation (see Chapter 8). However, the fact remains that BOLD is caused by neuronal activities in a complicated way called neurovascular coupling (NVC). Discovering the physiological details of NVC will greatly inform our understanding of the inner working of basic sensory system and higher cognitive functions.

One of the major obstacles against accessing neuronal activities is the spatial resolution of fMRI images that stood at about 50 mm^3 at 1.5 T. HF fMRI has improved BOLD resolution to about 1 mm^3 at 7 T. How could fMRI at such spatial resolution help investigate the brain's activity and response to external stimulation at a more basic level? One millimeter is the diameter of cortical columns and now experiments can be designed to detect functional activity at the columnar level and map functional connectivity of the cortical columns. Such possibilities are presently being explored [12,13]. The cerebral cortex is made up of basic functional units called cortical columns, which are lined up in a perpendicular direction to the cortical surface. Neurons in these vertical cluster share the same tuning for any given receptive field attribute. In order to enable fMRI to resolve cortical-columns level events, new acquisition and image analysis strategies are emerging, taking into account the fMRI point-spread, the voxel size, and the thermal and physiological noise. Point-spread function is a measure of spatial specificity of the BOLD response with the actual locus of neuronal activity. Work on finding the appropriate role of these factors will ultimately determine the optimum voxel size for studies using fMRI of cortical columns.

Future

Pushing the field strength of MRI scanners above 10 T will offer higher spatiotemporal resolution which could enable sufficient temporal signal-to-noise ratio (tSNR) needed for neuronal fMRI but will not come at a low cost. tSNR offers information on the data quality of fMRI time series. Higher tSNR will allow acquisition of data that more accurately represents neuronal activity (neuronal fMRI). Another technical limitation associated with magnetic susceptibilities across tissue/air boundaries that kills the MRI signal (causes signal drop outs) in brain regions in the vicinity of nasal cavity, paranasal sinuses, skull base, temporal bone, mastoid air cells, and middle ear cavities requires sophisticated solutions to ensure acquisition of homogeneous BOLD data over the whole brain. Other technical issues involve the penetration depth of the RF(B1 +) pulses, which makes the sensitivity of fMRI higher in the cortical regions compared with the thalamic regions. RF pulses used for excitation of spins, RF(B1 +), attenuate as they penetrate into the brain and as such their variation effects the quality of MRI images and its BOLD representation. This poses a serious challenge in fMRI studies involving the whole brain in subcortical structures for which high resolution is essential given their small sizes.

As field strength continues to increase, the SNR may improve sufficiently and decrease voxel size to the point where resolution is smaller than typical tissue movement within the voxel. As such, amplitude of microscopic motion limits the resolution of fMRI images. In such limits a combination of high spatiotemporal techniques could be applied to "freeze out" the cellular motion. HF challenges could be met by techniques such as adiabatic RF pulses, parallel transmit (pTx) B1 + shimming, 3D-echo planar imaging (EPI) signal readout, optimized parallel receive (pRx) acquisition and reconstruction, and optimized RF channel combination. Adiabatic RF pulses are the type of pulses that can excite spins uniformly in spite of the presence of RF inhomogeneities, which are a fact of life at HF, parallel transmit or pTx is capability of exciting multiple channels of an RF pulse at the same time, shimming with RF pulses rather than shim coils or B1 + shimming is a useful feature of multichannel coils that allow to produce more homogeneous images, acquisition of EPI in 3D rather than multislice mode is a capability that allows achievement of thinner slices and image reslicing postacquisition, parallel receive, or pRx is a capability of multichannel coils that help accelerate image acquisition and reduce scan time. Such solutions have already helped produce images with submillimeter spatial resolution of about 0.12 mm isotropic, i.e., voxels with the same dimension in all three directions, in a large field of view that has been reported at 7 T [14,15]. Once motion, susceptibility, and RF coil challenges are met, functional SNR could make BOLD mechanism more sensitive to the microvasculature [16] allowing it to more accurately locate the site of neuronal activity. Furthermore, it is conceivable that with new developments in multichannel RF coils [17] and simultaneous multislice excitation (SMS) technology [18,19], achieving much higher tSNR and temporal resolution fMRI is not far from reach. More advancements in parallel transmit [20,21] will further accelerate image acquisition allowing us to arrive at 0.1 mm^3/100 ms spatial/temporal resolution which will approach the speed of neuronal activity in the brain.

Conclusion

In summary, to reap the full benefits of HF MRI, a number of technical developments capable of addressing the difficulties of high field are within our reach. HF MRI is an important tool for future studies that can revolutionize investigation of brain structure and function and is presently standing at the threshold of detection of cortical microcircuitry in humans [22–25].

Beyond the brain: Toward an integrative cross-disciplinary understanding of human behavior and experience

27

Laurence J. Kirmayer

From the intricate drawings of dense forests of neurons by the great neuroanatomist Ramon y Cajal [1], to computer-generated animations of the shimmering circuitry of the human connectome [2], images of the brain captivate our imagination and seem to offer us a window into our essential nature. But pictures of the brain are not pictures of the mind. We need a much larger view than that provided by any brain scanner to get a glimpse of the systems that give rise to our feelings, thoughts, aspirations, sense of self, and personhood. To get even a rudimentary picture of the mind at work and at play, we need to capture not just the contents of the skull, but the texture of experience and the landscape of the worlds we live in—worlds that are made up of all sorts of things, most especially other people, who participate in the complex forms of cooperative activity we call "culture." The functioning of the brain can only be understood in relation to our transactions with the social-ecological niches we inhabit and making sense of this interaction requires more than imaging technology [3].

The brain evolved to allow human beings to live our very distinctive sorts of lives—endowed with consciousness and animated by restless imagination, creativity, and constant cultural innovation. Although physically vulnerable in many ways, we have migrated across the globe and learned to survive in very diverse and challenging environments, from the desert to the arctic. Our successes in adaptation have depended on the ways our brains allow us to work together to devise new technologies and build habitable environments. In the process, we have redefined ourselves as a species many times.

Culture and the brain, nature and nurture, interact on multiple time scales [3]. In the evolutionary emergence of *Homo sapiens*, changes in the anatomy of the brain—reflected in the deep corrugations of the neocortex and other structures—enabled our complex social behavior. We then constructed social worlds to which we have adapted in a process of brain-culture coevolution [4]. Culture reshapes the brain throughout development, switching genes on and off, remodeling neural architecture, and modulating synaptic transmission. All these forms of

Casting Light on the Dark Side of Brain Imaging. DOI: https://doi.org/10.1016/B978-0-12-816179-1.00027-X

neuroplasticity allow our brains to become attuned to the environments we inhabit. Culturally shaped modes of childrearing remodel our brains so that we can speak certain languages and decode the norms and contexts that allow us to function in social roles. Finally, we face everyday challenges adapting and improvising to specific demands created by our changing cultural worlds.

The brain makes culture possible and puts some general constraints on the forms of cultural life—but we can readily surpass them. We can see some of these elementary building blocks of cognition in the laboratory when we pose game-like puzzles to people to see how their brains are activated as they try to solve these tasks. We can get an inkling of other crucial building blocks of situated cognition when we employ novel approaches like scanning two people as they interact [5]. This kind of research can reveal modes of interpersonal interaction which are basic ingredients of sociality. Unfortunately, current scanning methods are limited in both the physical and temporal scales they can capture. As a result, they cannot capture many essential features of social and cultural cognition.

From the social-cultural perspective, though, triads are more basic than dyads—both because care for infants by more than one person is basic to the structure of

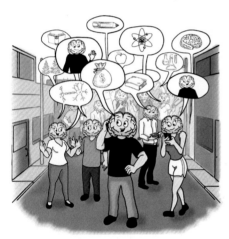

the family and, more broadly, because the interaction between two people always occurs against the backdrop of a larger social world, whether present in person, virtually in imagination, or implicitly in language and shared norms. The brain is designed to promote certain forms of social interaction like attachment and affiliation with those we perceive as emotionally close to us (like family, caregivers, or members of a social in-group) and wariness, fear or aggression against those we perceive as unfamiliar, strange, and threatening [6]. We readily and rapidly make these assignments to in-group and outgroup and respond accordingly. However, culturally mediated depictions of others can shift these assignments so that we come to respond to others with compassion and concern.

The essential lesson of cultural history and diversity is that, whatever evolution has given us in terms of the structures of the brain with which we think, we can reconfigure these in new and surprising ways that open up whole new landscapes of possibilities. Cultural gadgets and affordances allow us to use our brains in new and unanticipated ways [7,8]. The same visual acuity that allowed us to hunt for prey and avoid predators can be recruited to decode the markings on paper that open up endless possibilities of reading.

Human lives are lived with other people. We dwell in humanly designed ecological niches—populated with other people and shaped by cooperative action. This cooperation creates both the material constructions and the social institutions, values, and practices that allow us to define and pursue our goals. Indeed, in everyday thinking, we use this social environment to guide our action—in effect, we think *through* other minds [9].

A new model of the mind has emerged in recent years, which sees thinking as a process that occurs not only just in the neural "wetware" or circuitry of the brain, but also necessarily through our bodies and our interactions with the world [10]. The capabilities of our bodies—their shape, internal proceses mechanics, and dexterity—make possible certain forms of thinking. Our language is built up on a scaffolding of metaphors that begin with basic bodily experiences and that grows ever more complex and multilayered, allowing us to scale the heights of abstract thought. Because of this origin of thinking in bodily experience, there continues to be two-way traffic between our bodies and our thoughts. For example, when we are standing we tend to think more about balance than we do when we are sitting, because standing is literally a balancing act. And when we think uplifting thoughts, our posture changes to become more erect (just as, in contrast, when we feel discouraged or debased, we slump in a posture of dejection). Thinking influences the body and the body, in turn, shapes thinking in an ongoing cycle. These basic forms of *embodiment* provide the underpinning to thought and break down any hard division between thinking, feeling, perceiving, and acting.

Of course, our bodies dwell in a world that affords us specific opportunities for action. We can move around to locate things that are good to eat and to avoid danger. But our actions are not just determined by the raw materials of the environment. We use tools, language, and symbolic codes to transform our environment and, in so doing, present our brains with new possibilities for action. We can pick up a stone and use it to crack open a coconut or use one stone to chip another fashioning it into an axe, a spear, or an arrowhead good for hunting. We can sit down with others in a hunting party and plan our strategy. Human evolution is a story of inventing new forms of cooperation (and, along with that, perhaps inevitably, new forms of conflict).

The recognition that thought, feeling, perception, and action fit together in ongoing cycles has led to the development of current theories of *enactivism* based on the view that cognition is oriented toward action [11]. We think in order to act on the world to ensure our own survival and flourishing—and the survival and flourishing of others. Taken seriously, this enactive view of the brain means that we can best understand what the brain is doing by seeing how it functions in a particular context that includes the body and the environment. And human environments are both physical and *social*—that is to say, largely constituted by other people, each with their own bodies, brains, and expectations.

The mind then depends on the brain—not as a solo instrument, but playing in concert with other brains, whether following a score or improvising. Complex human thought is deeply cultural and historical—building on our shared history which is encoded in language, customs, rituals, practices, protocols—a whole way of life. These ways of life allow us to make use of the learning and experience of previous generations and our contemporaries. We need all of the social sciences and humanities, as well as an understanding of the dynamics of complex systems to begin to understand how our brains adapt to the environments we fashion.

To take one pivotal example, the forms of human thinking changed radically with the invention of writing and reading [12]. Being able to store detailed records and reminders of our thoughts and recipes for action and to reproduce and widely share this knowledge allowed a dramatic amplification of our powers of thought. The worlds' libraries are a vast storehouse of knowledge we can access and build on. This has expanded the temporal scale and scope of memory. We owe all of the remarkable advances of science to this capacity to extend our mind's vision and reach through forms of social interaction that draw from a common fund of knowledge, new technologies for exploring the world, and, especially, culturally grounded modes of critical thinking, argument, demonstration, and debate. Without a culturally based recognition of the epistemic authority of science, we risk living in a post-truth world in which "might makes right."

We are currently witnessing a further revolution in knowledge production and sharing through the use of computers and the Internet. We are now able to offload knowledge to digital media and share it globally. We can access knowledge from around the globe, at all levels of detail and expertise, instantaneously. As automatic translation methods improve, so will the scope of the available information and communication in real-time.

These technological advances herald a new expansion of the human mind—brain—body—person beyond the confines of the human skull. We can think together across long stretches of historical time and diverse cultures. This allows us to bring together the great diversity of ways of thinking developed by different language communities and cultures with cooperative action at many scales, from local groups that can arrange collective action, to globe spanning networks that can distribute tasks and coordinate large scale cooperation.

New forms of social cooperation create new possibilities for thought, new ways of using our brains and, with that, changes in our neural architecture based on developmental neuroplasticity and, eventually, evolution. The current environments to which we must adapt pose new challenges both in the scale, speed, density, and kinds of information to which we must respond. It is likely our brains will change in response to the new exigencies we are creating through technologies like the Internet, social media, and artificial intelligence.

Speculative fiction writers have imagined many possible "posthuman" worlds in which we are supplanted by our machines or become part of human-machine hybrids, living in virtual worlds. These scenarios range from hardware augmentation of the brain, to biological modifications of neural processing and cellular and molecular levels, to the integration of individuals into large networks of which our fleshly bodies are only a small and fungible part. Understanding the consequences of these forms of self-modification will require considering their impacts far beyond the functions of the brain itself.

Whatever our ultimate fate, we face important challenges to our survival at this moment. These challenges are closely related to the ways that we respond to others. A central question for our time is whether the forms of morality undergirded by a sense of belonging, mutual respect, compassion and care that worked for small local groups can be effectively extended to the much larger groups constituted by planetary networks. We need planetary thinking to support a global social ecosystem that allows humanity to continue to expand the reach of our minds. To devise ways to meet this challenge, it matters a great deal whether we see our modes of moral engagement as hard-wired into the brain or shaped by cultural values and practices over the course of development.

Additional readings

Kirmayer LJ. The future of critical neuroscience. In: Choudhury S, Slaby J, editors. Critical neuroscience: a handbook of the social and cultural contexts of neuroscience. New York: Wiley-Blackwell; 2012. p. 367−83.

Kirmayer LJ, Crafa D. What kind of science for psychiatry? Front Hum Neurosci 2014;8.

Kirmayer LJ. Re-visioning psychiatry: toward an ecology of mind in health and illness. Re-visioning psychiatry: cultural phenomenology, critical neuroscience and global mental health. New York: Cambridge University Press; 2015. p. 622−60.

Kirmayer LJ, Ramstead MJ. Embodiment and enactment in cultural psychiatry. In: Durt C, Fuchs T, editors. Embodiment, enaction, and culture: investigating the constitution of the shared world, 397. Cambrudge, MA: MIT Press; 2017.

Conclusion

Robert T. Thibault

Everything looks like a nail if all you have is a hammer. Or at least so the saying goes. In a nutshell, this was the main point we hoped to communicate. Hammers are good for nails. But to build a house, you need many tools.

The same goes for understanding human behavior and brain function. Neuroimaging is an important set of techniques toward this goal, but only one among many. Psychology, psychiatry, cognitive science, artificial intelligence, social studies, anthropology, and other levels of neuroscientific analysis such as single cells and neurotransmitters all have their role to play. Selecting our tools in light of a scientific question may better help progress than selecting a question based on the tools we are familiar with. Using diverse methods to triangulate evidence, moreover, can only help us arrive at a more scientific understanding of the questions that brain imaging aims to solve.

The brain has earned a central position in contemporary discourse about human behavior. Advances in neuroimaging techniques and the appealing reductionist story they tell have surely helped bring the brain to the fore. As with many young fields of research, we can display the progress of neuroimaging on the now popularized, and occasionally accurate, Gartner Hype Cycle (see image).

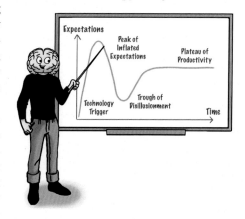

Currently, neuroimaging seems to land somewhere near the peak. If we asked a conference hall full of neuroscientists where on this graph they think brain imaging sits, we believe that most would agree with us. Where they would disagree, however, is on how to best move from the *peak of inflated expectations* to the *plateau of productivity*, without getting stuck in the *trough of disillusionment*. We prepared this volume, in part, with the hope to help smooth this transition. At the *peak*, scientists and the public over-accentuate neuroimaging research, and at times, use it in an attempt to answer questions where other methods would better serve us. At the *trough*, people have given up on brain imaging, even where it remains useful. Among the discussions this volume offered on the applications of neuroimaging, the methodological considerations, the shortcomings of neuroreductionism, and the future promises this field holds, we aimed to balance skepticism with breakthroughs: to squash hype and circumvent disillusionment.

We didn't prepare this volume to turn you into an expert brain imager. Instead, we compiled it to provide a broad base of knowledge that can help to identify the pitfalls as well as potential of neuroimaging. To help readers judiciously evaluate brain imaging findings. And to help you translate common sayings, such as "my brain made me do it," into the more cumbersome, yet more accurate, "my brain *within this body, surrounding environment, and social context* made me do it." The centrality of the brain in current discussions about human mental life is not in itself a problem, but treating the brain as the sole causal mechanism behind human action can sometimes miss the point. Pushing neuroimaging forward with rigorous methodologies, nuance, and skepticism can only help in uncovering what makes humans tick.

References

Neuroskepticism: questioning the brain as symbol and selling-point

[1] Poldrack RA, Mumford JA. Independence in ROI analysis: where is the voodoo? Soc Cogn Affect Neurosci 2009;4.2:208—13.
[2] Bennett CM, Miller MB, Wolford GL. Neural correlates of interspecies perspective taking in the post-mortem Atlantic Salmon: an argument for multiple comparisons correction. Neuroimage 2009;47(Suppl. 1):S125.
[3] Eklund A, Nichols TE, Knutsson H. Cluster failure: why fMRI inferences for spatial extent have inflated false-positive rates. Proc Natl Acad Sci USA 2016;113(28):7900—5.

Chapter 1

[1] Fodor J. Why, why, does everyone go on so about the brain? Lond Rev Books 1999;21 (19):68—9.
[2] Harnad S. To cognize is to categorize: cognition is categorization. In: Cohen H, Lefebvre C, editors. Handbook of categorization in cognitive science. 2nd ed. Elsevier; 2017.
[3] Turing AM. Computing machinery and intelligence. Mind 1950;59(236):433—60.
[4] Feigl H. The mind-body problem in the development of logical empiricism. Revue Internationale de Philosophie 1950;64—83.

Chapter 2

[1] Hume D, Hendel C, editors. An inquiry concerning human understanding. Indianapolis: Bobbs-Merrill; 1955.
[2] Atmanspacher H, Primas H. The hidden side of Wolfgang Pauli: an eminent physicist's extraordinary encounter with depth psychology. J Conscious Stud 1996;3:112—26.
[3] Popper K. The logic of scientific discovery. New York: Routledge; 2005.
[4] Leshner AI. Addiction is a brain disease, and it matters. Science 1997;278:45—7.
[5] Volkow ND, Koob GF, McLellan AT. Neurobiologic advances from the brain disease model of addiction. N Engl J Med 2016;374:363—71.
[6] Volkow ND, Koob G. Brain disease model of addiction: why is it so controversial? Lancet Psychiatry 2015;2:677—9.

[7] Botticelli MP, Koh HK. Changing the language of addiction. J Am Med Assoc 2016;316:1361−2.

[8] Drugs, brains, and behavior: the science of addiction. *National Institute on Drug Abuse*; 2014.

[9] Grifell M, Hart CL. Is drug addiction a brain disease? This popular claim lacks evidence and leads to poor policy. Am Sci 2018;106:160−7.

[10] Skeide MA, Kumar U, Mishra RK, Tripathi VN, Guleria A, Singh JP, et al. Learning to read alters cortico-subcortical cross-talk in the visual system of illiterates. Sci Adv 2017;3:e1602612.

[11] Draganski B, Gaser C, Busch V, Schuierer G, Bogdahn U, May A. Neuroplasticity: changes in grey matter induced by training. Nature 2004;427:311−12.

[12] Satel S, Lilienfeld SO. Brainwashed: the seductive appeal of mindless neuroscience. New York: Basic Books; 2013.

[13] Hart C. High price: a neuroscientist's journey of self-discovery that challenges everything you know about drugs and society. New York: Harper Collins Publishers; 2013.

[14] Lewis M. Addiction and the brain: development, not disease. Neuroethics 2017;10:7−18.

[15] Kendler KS. Toward a philosophical structure for psychiatry. Am J Psychiatr 2005;162:433−40.

[16] Satel S, Lilienfeld SO. Addiction and the brain-disease fallacy. Front Psychiatr 2014;4:141.

[17] Heyman GM. Addiction and choice: theory and new data. Front Psychiatr 2013;4:31.

[18] Heyman GM, Lilienfeld SO, Morse S, Satel S. Brief of Amici Curiae of 11 addiction experts in support of appellee. University of Pennsylvania Law School, Public Law Research Paper No. 17-44; 2018.

[19] Cohen P, Cohen J. The clinician's illusion. Arch Gen Psychiatr 1984;41:1178−82.

[20] Robins LN, Davis DH, Nurco DN. How permanent was Vietnam drug addiction? Am J Public Health 1974;64:38−43.

[21] George WH, Gilmore AK, Stappenbeck CA. Balanced placebo design: revolutionary impact on addictions research and theory. Addict Res Theory 2012;20:186−203.

[22] Lilienfeld SO. Clinical psychological science: then and now. Clin Psychol Sci 2017;5:3−13.

[23] Hall W, Carter A, Forlini C. The brain disease model of addiction: is it supported by the evidence and has it delivered on its promises? Lancet Psychiatry 2015;2:105−10.

[24] Kellogg SH, Stitzer ML, Petry NM, Kreek MJ. Contingency management: foundations and principles. Natl Inst Drug Abuse 2007.

[25] Prendergast M, Podus D, Finney J, Greenwell L, Roll J. Contingency management for treatment of substance use disorders: a meta-analysis. Addiction 2006;101:1546−60.

[26] Trujols J. The brain disease model of addiction: challenging or reinforcing stigma? Lancet Psychiatry 2015;2:292.

[27] Graham C. Happiness for all? Unequal lives and hopes in pursuit of the American dream. Princeton: *Princeton University Press*; 2017.

[28] Satel S, Lilienfeld SO. Calling addition a 'brain disease' makes it harder to treat. Boston Globe; 2017.

Chapter 3

[1] Vigo D, Thornicroft G, Atun R. Estimating the true global burden of mental illness. Lancet Psychiatry 2016;3:171−8.
[2] Hyde TM, Weinberger DR. The brain in schizophrenia. Semin Neurol 1990;10:276−86.
[3] Frances A. The past, present and future of psychiatric diagnosis. World Psychiatry 2013;12:111−12.
[4] Huber G. The pneumoencephalogram at the onset of schizophrenic disease. Arch Psychiatr Nervenkr Z Gesamte Neurol Psychiatr 1955;193:406−26.
[5] Witkowski M, et al. Mapping entrained brain oscillations during transcranial alternating current stimulation (tACS). Neuroimage 2016;140:89−98.
[6] Chander BS, et al. tACS phase locking of frontal midline theta oscillations disrupts working memory performance. Front Cell Neurosci 2016;10:120.
[7] Ushiba J, Soekadar SR. Brain-machine interfaces for rehabilitation of poststroke hemiplegia. Prog Brain Res 2016;228:163−83.
[8] Braun U, et al. From maps to multi-dimensional network mechanisms of mental disorders. Neuron 2018;97:14−31.

Chapter 4

[1] Norris FH. Amyotrophic lateral sclerosis: the clinical disorder. Handbook of amyotrophic lateral sclerosis. 1992. p. 3−38.
[2] Bensch M, Martens S, Halder S, Hill J, Nijboer F, Ramos A, et al. Assessing attention and cognitive function in completely locked-in state with event-related brain potentials and epidural electrocorticography. J Neural Eng 2014;11(2).
[3] Birbaumer N, Ghanayim N, Hinterberger T, Iversen I, Kotchoubey B, Kübler A, et al. A spelling device for the paralysed. Nature 1999;398:297−8.
[4] Birbaumer N, Cohen LG. Brain−computer-interfaces (BCI): communication and restoration of movement in paralysis. J Physiol 2007.
[5] Massari DD, Ruf CA, Furdea A, Matuz T, Heiden L, Halder S, et al. Brain communication in the locked-in state. Brain 2013;136:1989−2000.
[6] Kübler A, Birbaumer N. Brain−computer interfaces and communication in paralysis: extinction of goal directed thinking in completely paralysed patients? Clin Neurophysiol 2008;119:2658−66.
[7] Ramos A, Hill J, Bensch M, Martens S, Halder S, Nijboer F, et al. Transition from the locked in to the completely locked-in State: a physiological analysis. Clin Neurophysiol 2011;122:925−33.
[8] Hochberg LR, Serruya MD, Friehs GM, Mukand JA, Saleh M, Caplan AH, et al. Neuronal ensemble control of prosthetic devices by a human with tetraplegia. Nature 2006;442:164−71.
[9] Hochberg LR, Bacher D, Jarosiewicz B, Masse NY, Simeral JD, Vogel J, et al. Reach and grasp by people with tetraplegia using a neurally controlled robotic arm. Nature 2012;485(7398):372−5.
[10] Birbaumer N, Piccione F, Silvoni S, Wildgruber M. Ideomotor silence: the case of complete paralysis and brain−computer interfaces (BCI). Psychol Res 2012;76:183−91.

[11] Dworkin BR, Miller NE. Failure to replicate visceral learning in the acute curarized rat preparation. Behav Neurosci 1986;100(3):299–314.
[12] Dworkin BR. Learning and physiological regulation. Chicago: University of Chicago Press; 1993.
[13] Gallegos-Ayala G, Furdea A, Takano K, Ruf CA, Flor H, Birbaumer N. Brain communication in a completely locked-in patient using bedside near-infrared spectroscopy. Neurology 2014;82:1–3.
[14] Birbaumer N, Ruiz S, Sitaram R. Learned regulation of brain metabolism. Trends Cogn Sci TICS 2013;17(6):295–302.
[15] Chaudhary U, Xia B, Silvoni S, Cohen LG, Birbaumer N. Brain–computer interface-based communication in the completely locked-in state. PLoS Biol 2017;15:1.
[16] Naito M, Michioka Y, Ozawa K, Ito Y, Kiguchi M, Kanazawa T. A communication means for totally locked-in ALS patients based on changes in cerebral blood volume measured with near-infrared light. IEICE Trans Inf Syst 2007;E90-D(7):1028–37.
[17] Guger C, Spataro R, Allison BZ, Heilinger A, Ortner R, Cho W, et al. Complete locked-in and locked-in patients: command following assessment and communication with vibro-tactile P300 and motor imagery brain–computer interface tools. Front Neurosci 2017;11:251.
[18] Chaudhary U, Birbaumer N, Ramos A. Brain–computer interface for communication and rehabilitation. Nat Rev Neurol 2016;12(9):513–25.

Chapter 5

[1] The Economist. The ethics of brain sciences: open your mind; 2002 [cited 2018 Jan 17]. Available from: <www.economist.com/node/1143317/print> May 23 [Internet].
[2] Morse SJ. Brain overclaim syndrome: a diagnostic note. Ohio State J Crim Law 2006;3(2):397–412.
[3] Morse SJ. Brain overclaim redux. Law Inequal 2013;31(2):509–34.
[4] Morse SJ. Lost in translation? An essay on law and neuroscience. In: Freeman M, editor. Law Neurosci 2011;13(28):529–62.
[5] Mudrik L, Maoz U. "Me & my brain": exposing neuroscience's closet dualism. J Cogn Neurosci 2015;27(2):211–21.
[6] Morse SJ. The non-problem of free will in forensic psychiatry and psychology. Behav Sci Law 2007;25(2):203–20.
[7] Greene J, Cohen J. For the law, neuroscience changes nothing and everything. In: Zeki S, Goodenough O, editors. Law and the brain. New York: Oxford University Press; 2006. p. 1775–85.
[8] Adolph R. The unsolved problems of neuroscience. Trends Cogn Sci 2015;19(4):173–5.
[9] McHugh PR, Slavney PR. The perspectives of psychiatry. 2nd ed Baltimore: Johns Hopkins University Press; 1998. p. 352.
[10] Morse SJ. Oxford handbooks online [Internet]. Oxford: Oxford University Press; 2017. Neuroethics: neurolaw. Available from: http://www.oxfordhandbooks.com/view/10.1093/oxfordhb/9780199935314.001.0001/oxfordhb-9780199935314-e-45?print = pdf.
[11] Morse SJ, Newsome WT. Criminal responsibility, criminal competence, and prediction of criminal behavior. In: Morse SJ, Roskies AL, editors. A primer on criminal law and neuroscience. New York: Oxford University Press; 2013. p. 150–78.

[12] Greely HT. Mind reading, neuroscience, and the law. In: Morse SJ, Roskies AL, editors. A primer on criminal law and neuroscience. New York: Oxford University Press; 2013. p. 120−49.

[13] Husak D, Murphy E. The relevance of the neuroscience of addiction to the criminal law. In: Morse SJ, Roskies AL, editors. A primer on criminal law and neuroscience. New York: Oxford University Press; 2013. p. 216−39.

[14] Aharoni E, Vincent GM, Harenski CL, Calhoun VD, Sinnott-Armstrong W, Gazzaniga MS, et al. Neuroprediction of future rearrest. Proc Natl Acad Sci 2013;110 (15):6223−8.

[15] Vilares I, Wesley MJ, Ahn WY, Bonnie RJ, Hoffman M, Jones OD, et al. Predicting the knowledge−recklessness distinction in the human brain. Proc Natl Acad Sci USA 2017;114(12):3222−7.

[16] Pustilnik AC. Imaging brains, changing minds: how pain neuroimaging can help transform the law. Alabama Law Rev 2015;66(5):1099−158.

Chapter 6

[1] Bruer JT. Education and the brain: a bridge too far. Educ Res 1997;26(8):4−16.

[2] Horvath JC, Donoghue GM. A bridge too far−revisited: reframing Bruer's neuroeducation argument for modern science of learning practitioners. Front Psychol 2016;7:377.

[3] Donoghue GM, Horvath JC. Translating neuroscience, psychology and education: an abstracted conceptual framework for the learning sciences. Cogent Educ 2016;3 (1):1267422.

[4] Bowers JS. The practical and principled problems with educational neuroscience. Psychol Rev 2016;123(5):600.

[5] Okano H, Hirano T, Balaban E. Learning and memory. Proc Natl Acad Sci USA 2000;97(23):12403−4.

[6] Mayer RE. Learning and instruction. Prentice Hall; 2003.

[7] Shuell TJ. Cognitive conceptions of learning. Rev Educ Res 1986;56(4):411−36. p. 412.

[8] Hebb DO. The organization of behavior: a neuropsychological theory; 1949.

[9] Colvin R. Optimising, generalising and integrating educational practice using neuroscience. NPJ Sci Learn 2016;1:16012.

[10] Levitin DJ. This is your brain on music: the science of a human obsession. Penguin; 2006.

[11] Perry BD. Childhood experience and the expression of genetic potential: what childhood neglect tells us about nature and nurture. Brain Mind 2002;3 (1):79−100.

[12] Weisberg DS, Keil FC, Goodstein J, Rawson E, Gray JR. The seductive allure of neuroscience explanations. J Cogn Neurosci 2008;20(3):470−7.

[13] Donoghue GM. Translating neuroscience and psychology into education: towards a conceptual model for the science of learning. Unpublished doctoral thesis, University of Melbourne; 2017.

[14] Bruer JT. Building bridges in neuroeducation. Educ Brain Essays Neuroeduc 2008;43−58.

[15] Schroder HS, Moran TP, Donnellan MB, Moser JS. Mindset induction effects on cognitive control: a neurobehavioral investigation. Biol Psychol 2014;103:27−37.
[16] Moser JS. How Your Brain Reacts To Mistakes Depends On Your Mindset. Association for Psychological Science 2011. From: <https://www.psychologicalscience.org/news/releases/how-the-brain-reacts-to-mistakes.html>.
[17] Schroder HS, Moran TP, Donnellan MB, Moser JS. Mindset induction effects on cognitive control: a neurobehavioral investigation. Biol Psychol 2014;103:35.
[18] Boaler J. Mistakes grow your brain; 2017. From <https://www.youcubed.org/evidence/mistakes-grow-brain/> [accessed 29.11.17].
[19] Science of Learning Research Centre, <https://www.slrc.org.au/resources/pen-principles/>.

Chapter 7

[1] Gray CM, Singer W. Stimulus-specific neuronal oscillations in orientation columns of cat visual-cortex. Proc Natl Acad Sci USA 1989;86(5):1698−702.
[2] Yuval-Greenberg S, Tomer O, Keren AS, Nelken I, Deouelll LY. Transient induced gamma-band response in EEG as a manifestation of miniature saccades. Neuron 2008;58 (3):429−41.
[3] Whitham EM, Pope KJ, Fitzgibbon SP, Lewis T, Clark CR, Loveless S, et al. Scalp electrical recording during paralysis: quantitative evidence that EEG frequencies above 20 Hz are contaminated by EMG. Clin Neurophysiol 2007;118(8):1877−88.
[4] Millett D. Hans Berger: from psychic energy to the EEG. Perspect Biol Med 2001;44 (4):522−42.

Chapter 8

[1] Kwong KK, Belliveau JW, Chesler DA, Goldberg IE, Weisskoff RM, Poncelet BP, et al. Dynamic magnetic resonance imaging of human brain activity during primary sensory stimulation. Proc Natl Acad Sci USA 1992;89:5675−9.
[2] Ogawa S, Tank DW, Menon R, Ellermann JM, Kim SG, Merkle H, et al. Intrinsic signal changes accompanying sensory stimulation: functional brain mapping with magnetic-resonance-imaging. Proc Natl Acad Sci USA 1992;89:5951−5.
[3] Bandettini PA, Wong EC, Hinks RS, Tikofsky RS, Hyde JS. Time course EPI of human brain function during task activation. Magn Reson Med 1992;25:390−7.
[4] Ogawa S, Lee TM, Kay AR, Tank DW. Brain magnetic resonance imaging with contrast dependent on blood oxygenation. Proc Natl Acad Sci USA 1990;87:9868−72.
[5] Fox PT, Raichle ME. Focal physiological uncoupling of cerebral blood-flow and oxidative-metabolism during somatosensory stimulation in human-subjects. Proc Natl Acad Sci USA 1986;83:1140−4.
[6] Hoge RD, Atkinson J, Gill B, Crelier GR, Marrett S, Pike GB. Linear coupling between cerebral blood flow and oxygen consumption in activated human cortex. Proc Natl Acad Sci USA 1999;96:9403−8.
[7] Buxton RB, Uludag K, Dubowitz DJ, Liu TT. Modeling the hemodynamic response to brain activation. NeuroImage 2004;23:S220−33.

[8] Lu H, van Zijl PC. A review of the development of vascular-space-occupancy (VASO) fMRI. NeuroImage 2003;62:736–42.

[9] Mathiesen C, Caesar K, Akgoren N, Lauritzen M. Modification of activity dependent increases of cerebral blood flow by excitatory synaptic activity and spikes in rat cerebellar cortex. J Physiol (Lond) 1998;512:555–66.

[10] Heeger DJ, Huk AC, Geisler WS, Albrecht DG. Spikes versus BOLD: what does neuroimaging tell us about neuronal activity? Nat Neurosci 2000;3:631–3.

[11] Logothetis NK, Pauls J, Augath M, Trinath T, Oeltermann A. Neurophysiological investigation of the basis of the fMRI signal. Nature 2001;412:150–7.

[12] Smith AJ, Blumenfeld H, Behar KL, Rothman DL, Shulman RG, Hyder F. Cerebral energetics and spiking frequency: the neurophysiological basis of fMRI. Proc Natl Acad Sci USA 2002;99:10765–70.

[13] Devor A, Dunn AK, Andermann ML, Ulbert I, Boas DA, Dale AM. Coupling of total hemoglobin concentration, oxygenation, and neural activity in rat somatosensory cortex. Neuron 2003;39:353–9.

[14] Jones M, Hewson-Stoate N, Martindale J, Redgrave P, Mayhew J. Nonlinear coupling of neural activity and CBF in rodent barrel cortex. NeuroImage 2004;22:956–65.

[15] Sheth SA, Nemoto M, Guiou M, Walker M, Pouratian N, Toga AW. Linear and nonlinear relationships between neuronal activity, oxygen metabolism, and hemodynamic responses. Neuron 2004;42:347–55.

[16] Niessing J, Ebisch B, Schmidt KE, Niessing M, Singer W, Galuske RA. Hemodynamic signals correlate tightly with synchronized gamma oscillations. Science 2005;309:948–51.

[17] Saad ZS, Ropella KM, DeYoe EA, Bandettini PA. The spatial extent of the BOLD response. NeuroImage 2003;19:132–44.

[18] Engel SA, Glover GH, Wandell BA. Retinotopic organization in human visual cortex and the spatial precision of functional MRI. Cereb Cortex 1997;7:181–92.

[19] Shmuel A, Yacoub E, Chaimow D, Logothetis NK, Ugurbil K. Spatio-temporal point-spread function of fMRI signal in human gray matter at 7 Tesla. NeuroImage 2007;35:539–52.

[20] Chaimow D, Yacoub E, Uğurbil K, Shmuel A. Spatial specificity of the functional MRI blood oxygenation response relative to neuronal activity. NeuroImage 2018;164:32–47.

[21] Poplawsky AJ, Kim SG. Layer-dependent BOLD and CBV-weighted fMRI responses in the rat olfactory bulb. NeuroImage 2014;91:237–51.

[22] Huber L, Handwerker DA, Jangraw DC, Chen G, Hall A, Stüber C, et al. High-resolution CBV-fMRI allows mapping of laminar activity and connectivity of cortical input and output in human M1. Neuron 2017;96:1253–63.

[23] Fox MD, Raichle ME. Spontaneous fluctuations in brain activity observed with functional magnetic resonance imaging. Nat Rev Neurosci 2007;8:700–11.

[24] Shmuel A, Leopold DA. Neuronal correlates of spontaneous fluctuations in fMRI signals in monkey visual cortex: implications for functional connectivity at rest. Hum Brain Mapp 2008;29:751–61.

[25] Schölvinck M, Maier A, Ye F, Duyn J, Leopold DA. Neural basis of global resting-state fMRI activity. Proc Natl Acad Sci USA 2010;107:10238–43.

[26] Maier A, Wilke M, Aura C, Zhu C, Ye FQ, Leopold DA. Divergence of fMRI and neural signals in V1 during perceptual suppression in the awake monkey. Nat Neurosci 2008;11:1193–200.

[27] Sirotin YB, Das A. Anticipatory haemodynamic signals in sensory cortex not predicted by local neuronal activity. Nature 2009;457:475–9.

Chapter 9

[1] Kahn RS, Sommer IE. The neurobiology and treatment of first-episode schizophrenia. Mol Psychiatry 2015;20:84−97.

[2] Kühn S, Gallinat J. Brain structure and functional connectivity associated with pornography consumption: the brain on porn. JAMA Psychiatry 2014;71:827−34.

[3] Weinberger DR, Radulescu E. Finding the elusive psychiatric 'lesion' with 21st-century neuroanatomy: a note of caution. Am J Psychiatry 2016;173:27−33.

[4] Eklund A, Nichols TE, Knutsson H. Cluster failure: why fMRI inferences for spatial extent have inflated false-positive rates. Proc Natl Acad Sci USA 2016;113 201602413.

[5] Kastrup A, Krüger G, Glover GH, Moseley ME. Assessment of cerebral oxidative metabolism with breath holding and fMRI. Magn Reson Med 1999;42:608−11.

[6] Abbott DF, Opdam HI, Briellmann RS, Jackson GD. Brief breath holding may confound functional magnetic resonance imaging studies. Hum Brain Mapp 2005;24:284−90.

[7] Thomason ME, Burrows BE, Gabrieli JDE, Glover GH. Breath holding reveals differences in fMRI BOLD signal in children and adults. Neuroimage 2005;25:824−37.

[8] Birn RM, Diamond JB, Smith MA, Bandettini PA. Separating respiratory-variation-related fluctuations from neuronal-activity-related fluctuations in fMRI. Neuroimage 2006;31:1536−48.

[9] Birn RM, Smith Ma, Jones TB, Bandettini Pa. The respiration response function: the temporal dynamics of fMRI signal fluctuations related to changes in respiration. Neuroimage 2008;40:644−54.

Chapter 10

[1] Goodenough DR, Oltman PK, Sigman E, Cox PW. The rod-and-frame illusion in erect and supine observers. Percept Psychophys 1981;29:365−70.

[2] Caldwell JA, Prazinko B, Caldwell JL. Body posture affects electroencephalographic activity and psychomotor vigilance task performance in sleep-deprived subjects. Clin Neurophysiol 2003;114:23−31.

[3] Fardo F, Spironelli C, Angrilli A. Horizontal body position reduces cortical pain-related processing: evidence from late ERPs. PLoS One 2013;8:1−12.

[4] Lundström JN, Boyle JA, Jones-Gotman M. Body position-dependent shift in odor percept present only for perithreshold odors. Chem Senses 2008;33:23−33.

[5] Harmon-Jones E, Price TF, Harmon-Jones C. Supine body posture decreases rationalizations: testing the action-based model of dissonance. J Exp Soc Psychol 2015;56:228−34.

[6] Rosenbaum D, Mama Y, Algom D. Stand by your stroop: standing up enhances selective attention and cognitive control. Psychol Sci 2017; 095679761772127.

[7] Lipnicki DM, Byrne DG. Thinking on your back: solving anagrams faster when supine than when standing. Brain Res Cogn Brain Res 2005;24:719−22.

[8] Badr C, Elkins MR, Ellis ER. The effect of body position on maximal expiratory pressure and flow. Aust J Physiother 2002;48:95−102.

[9] Cole RJ. Postural baroreflex stimuli may affect EEG arousal and sleep in humans. J Appl Physiol 1989;67:2369−75.

[10] Jones A, Dean E. Body position change and its effect on hemodynamic and metabolic status. Hear Lung 2004;33:281–90.

[11] Kräuchi K, Cajochen C, Wirz-Justice A. A relationship between heat loss and sleepiness: effects of postural change and melatonin administration. J Appl Physiol 1997;83 (1):134–9.

[12] Alperin N, Hushek SG, Lee SH, Sivaramakrishnan A, Lichtor T. MRI study of cerebral blood flow and CSF flow dynamics in an upright posture: the effect of posture on the intracranial compliance and pressure. Acta Neurochir Suppl 2005;95:177–81.

[13] Di X, Kannurpatti SS, Rypma B, Biswal BB. Calibrating BOLD fMRI activations with neurovascular and anatomical constraints. Cereb Cortex 2013;23:255–63.

[14] Spironelli C, Busenello J, Angrilli A. Supine posture inhibits cortical activity: evidence from Delta and Alpha EEG bands. Neuropsychologia 2016;89:125–31.

[15] Lifshitz M, Thibault RT, Roth R, Raz A. Source-localization of brain states associated with canonical neuroimaging postures. J Cogn Neurosci 2017; in press.

[16] Rice JK, Rorden C, Little JS, Parra LC. Subject position affects EEG magnitudes. Neuroimage 2013;64:476–84.

[17] Benvenuti SM, Bianchin M, Angrilli A. Posture affects emotional responses: a head down bed rest and ERP study. Brain Cogn 2013;82:313–18.

[18] Ramon C, Schimpf PH, Haueisen J. Influence of head models on EEG simulations and inverse source localizations. Biomed Eng Online 2006;5:10.

[19] de Lange FP, Helmich RC, Toni I. Posture influences motor imagery: an fMRI study. Neuroimage 2006;33:609–17.

[20] Kano C. An ecological theory of motion sickness and postural instability an ecological theory of motion sickness and postural instability. Ecol Psychol 1991;3:241–52.

[21] Harmon-Jones E, Peterson CK. Supine body position reduces neural response to anger evocation. Psychol Sci 2009;20:1209–10.

[22] Ferri F, Busiello M, Campione GC, et al. The eye contact effect in request and emblematic hand gestures. Eur J Neurosci 2014;39:841–51.

[23] Stopczynski A, Stahlhut C, Larsen JE, Petersen MK, Hansen LK. The smartphone brain scanner: a portable real-time neuroimaging system. PLoS One 2014;9.

Chapter 11

[1] Collaboration OS. Estimating the reproducibility of psychological science. Science 2015;349(6251).

[2] Cremers HR, Wager TD, Yarkoni T. The relation between statistical power and inference in fMRI. PLoS One. 2017;12(11):1–20.

[3] Murphy K, Birn RM, Bandettini PA. Resting-state fMRI confounds and cleanup. Neuroimage 2013;80:349–59.

[4] Eklund A, Nichols TE, Knutsson H. Cluster failure: why fMRI inferences for spatial extent have inflated false-positive rates; 2016.

[5] Algermissen J, Mehler DMA. May the power be with you: are there highly powered studies in neuroscience, and how can we get more of them? J Neurophysiol 2018;119:2114–17.

[6] Ware JJ, Munafò MR. Significance chasing in research practice: causes, consequences and possible solutions. Addiction 2015;110(1):4–8.

[7]   Thornton A, Lee P. Publication bias in meta-analysis: its causes and consequences. J Clin Epidemiol 2000;53(2):207−16.

[8]   Ramsey S, Scoggins J. Practicing on the tip of an information iceberg? Evidence of underpublication of registered clinical trials in oncology. Oncologist. 2008;13 (9):925.

[9]   Simmons JP, Nelson LD, Simonsohn U. False-positive psychology: undisclosed flexibility in data collection and analysis allows presenting anything as significant. Psychol Sci 2011;22(11):1359−66.

[10] Carp J. On the plurality of (methodological) worlds: estimating the analytic flexibility of fMRI experiments. Front Neurosci 2012;6:149.

[11] Poldrack RA, Baker CI, Durnez J, et al. Scanning the horizon: towards transparent and reproducible neuroimaging research. Nat Rev Neurosci 2017;18(2):115−26.

[12] Ioannidis JPA. Why most discovered true associations are inflated. Epidemiology. 2008;19(5):640−8.

[13] Higginson AD, Munafò MR. Current incentives for scientists lead to underpowered studies with erroneous conclusions. PLoS Biol 2016;14(11):e2000995.

[14] Chambers CD. Registered reports: a new publishing initiative at cortex. Cortex 2013;49 (3):609−10.

[15] Jia X, Zhao N, Barton B, Burciu R, Carrière N, Cerasa A. Small effect size leads to reproducibility failure in resting-state fMRI studies; 2018:1−15.

[16] Bowring A, Maumet C, Nichols T. Exploring the impact of analysis software on task fMRI results. bioRxiv 2018.

[17] Brembs B. Prestigious science journals struggle to reach even average reliability. Front Hum Neurosci 2018;12(February):1−7.

[18] Nichols TE, Das S, Eickhoff SB, et al. Best practices in data analysis and sharing in neuroimaging using MRI. Nat Neurosci 2017;20(3):299−303.

[19] Turner BO, Paul EJ, Miller MB, Barbey AK. Small sample sizes reduce the replicability of task-based fMRI studies. Commun Biol 2018.

[20] Munafò MR, Smith GD. Repeating experiments is not enough. Nature 2018;553:399−401.

Chapter 12

[1]   Ioannidis JP. Why most published research findings are false. PLoS Med 2005;2(8): e124.

[2]   Button KS, Ioannidis JP, Mokrysz C, Nosek BA, Flint J, Robinson ES, et al. Power failure: why small sample size undermines the reliability of neuroscience. Nat Rev Neurosci 2013;14(5):365−76.

[3]   Yarkoni T. Big correlations in little studies: inflated fMRI correlations reflect low statistical power-commentary on Vul et al. (2009). Perspect Psychol Sci 2009;4(3):294−8.

[4]   Gelman A, Carlin J. Beyond power calculations: assessing Type S (sign) and Type M (magnitude) errors. Perspect Psychol Sci 2014;9(6):641−51.

[5]   Nord CL, Valton V, Wood J, Roiser JP. Power-up: a reanalysis of 'power failure' in neuroscience using mixture modeling. J Neurosci 2017;37(34):8051−61.

[6]   Dumas-Mallet E, Button KS, Boraud T, Gonon F, Munafo MR. Low statistical power in biomedical science: a review of three human research domains. R Soc Open Sci 2017;4(2):160254.

[7] Poldrack RA, Baker CI, Durnez J, Gorgolewski KJ, Matthews PM, Munafo MR, et al. Scanning the horizon: towards transparent and reproducible neuroimaging research. Nat Rev Neurosci 2017;18(2):115–26.

[8] David SP, Ware JJ, Chu IM, Loftus PD, Fusar-Poli P, Radua J, et al. Potential reporting bias in fMRI studies of the brain. PloS One 2013;8(7):e70104.

[9] Cremers HR, Wager TD, Yarkoni T. The relation between statistical power and inference in fMRI. PloS One 2017;12(11):e0184923.

[10] Geuter S, Lindquist MA, Wager TD. In: Cacioppo JT, Tassinary LG, Berntson GG, editors. Fundamentals of functional neuroimaging. Cambridge: Cambridge University Press; 2017.

[11] van Ast VA, Spicer J, Smith EE, Schmer-Galunder S, Liberzon I, Abelson JL, et al. Brain mechanisms of social threat effects on working memory. Cereb Cortex 2016;26 (2):544–56.

[12] Yarkoni T, Poldrack RA, Nichols TE, Van Essen DC, Wager TD. Large-scale automated synthesis of human functional neuroimaging data. Nat Methods 2011;8 (8):665–70.

[13] Eisenbarth H, Chang LJ, Wager TD. Multivariate brain prediction of heart rate and skin conductance responses to social threat. J Neurosci 2016;36(47):11987–98.

[14] Yeo BT, Krienen FM, Sepulcre J, Sabuncu MR, Lashkari D, Hollinshead M, et al. The organization of the human cerebral cortex estimated by intrinsic functional connectivity. J Neurophysiol 2011;106(3):1125–65.

[15] Woo CW, Chang LJ, Lindquist MA, Wager TD. Building better biomarkers: brain models in translational neuroimaging. Nat Neurosci 2017;20(3):365–77.

[16] Reddan MC, Lindquist MA, Wager TD. Effect size estimation in neuroimaging. JAMA Psychiatry 2017;74(3):207–8.

[17] Wager TD, Atlas LY, Lindquist MA, Roy M, Woo CW, Kross E. An fMRI-based neurologic signature of physical pain. N Engl J Med 2013;368(15):1388–97.

[18] Krishnan A, Woo CW, Chang LJ, Ruzic L, Gu X, Lopez-Sola M, et al. Somatic and vicarious pain are represented by dissociable multivariate brain patterns. eLife. 2016;5.

[19] Chang LJ, Gianaros PJ, Manuck SB, Krishnan A, Wager TD. A sensitive and specific neural signature for picture-induced negative affect. PLoS Biol 2015;13(6):e1002180.

[20] Lopez-Sola M, Koban L, Krishnan A, Wager TD. When pain really matters: a vicarious-pain brain marker tracks empathy for pain in the romantic partner. Neuropsychologia 2017.

Chapter 13

[1] Orrù G, Pettersson-Yeo W, Marquand AF, Sartori G, Mechelli A. Using support vector machine to identify imaging biomarkers of neurological and psychiatric disease: a critical review. Neurosci Biobehav Rev 2012;36:1140–52.

[2] Mlodinow L. The drunkard's walk: how randomness rules our lives. Vintage; 2009.

[3] Baio J, Wiggins L, Christensen DL, Maenner MJ, Daniels J, Warren Z, et al. Prevalence of autism spectrum disorder among children aged 8 years—autism and developmental disabilities monitoring network, 11 sites, United States, 2014. MMWR Surveill Summar 2018;67(6):1.

[4] Autism and Developmental Disabilities Monitoring Network Surveillance Year 2010 Principal Investigators. Prevalence of autism spectrum disorder among children aged 8

years—autism and developmental disabilities monitoring network, 11 sites, United States, 2010. MMWR Surveill Summar 2014;63(2):1−21.

[5] Ecker C, Marquand A, Mourão-Miranda J, Johnston P, Daly EM, Brammer MJ, et al. Describing the brain in autism in five dimensions—magnetic resonance imaging-assisted diagnosis of autism spectrum disorder using a multiparameter classification approach. J Neurosci 2010;30(32):10612−23.

[6] Heneghan C. Why autism can't be diagnosed with brain scans. Guardian; 2010.

Chapter 14

[1] Nagel E. The structure of science. 2nd ed. Indianapolis: Hackett Publishing; 1979.

[2] Churchland PM. Eliminative materialism and the propositional attitudes. J Philos 1981;78(2):67−90.

[3] Churchland PM, Churchland PS. Interthreoretic reduction: a neuroscientist's field guide. In: Warner R, Szubka T, editors. The mind-body problem. Oxford: Blackwell; 1994.

[4] Barlow H. Single units and sensation: a neuron doctrine for perceptual psychology? Perception 1972;1(4):371−94.

[5] Maudlin T. On the unification of physics. J Philos 1996;93(3):129−44.

Chapter 15

[1] Horikawa T, Kamitani Y. Generic decoding of seen and imagined objects using hierarchical visual features. Nat Commun 2017;8:15037.

[2] McCabe DP, Castel AD. Seeing is believing: the effect of brain images on judgments of scientific reasoning. Cognition 2008;107:343−52.

[3] Olson JA, Landry M, Appourchaux K, Raz A. Simulated thought insertion: influencing the sense of agency using deception and magic. Conscious Cogn 2016;43:11−26.

[4] Ali SS, Lifshitz M, Raz A. Empirical neuroenchantment: from reading minds to thinking critically. Front Hum Neurosci 2014.

Chapter 16

[1] Ali SS, Lifshitz M, Raz A. Empirical neuroenchantment: from reading minds to thinking critically. Front Hum Neurosci 2014;8.

[2] Olson JA, Landry M, Appourchaux K, Raz A. Simulated thought insertion: influencing the sense of agency using deception and magic. Conscious Cogn 2016;43:11−26.

[3] Veissière S, Olson J, Raz A. Open-label suggestion improves self-regulation in neurodevelopmental disorders: a feasibility study. In: Poster presented at the 68th annual meeting of the society for clinical and experimental hypnosis, Chicago, IL, October 29, 2017.

[4] Thibault RT, Veissière S, Olson JA, Raz A. Treating ADHD with suggestion: neuro-feedback and placebo therapeutics. J Atten Disord 2018.

[5] RDoC is a new research framework developed by the National Institute of Mental Health to replace the Diagnostic and Statistical Manual of Mental Disorders (DSM). The RDoC aims to study mental disorders on multiple levels (from genetic to self-report), but is primarily focused on molecular and brain-based understandings of mental illness.

[6] Centers for Disease Control and Prevention. Attention-deficit/hyperactivity disorder (ADHD) [Internet]; 2017 [cited 2018 Jan 22]. Available from: <https://www.cdc.gov/ncbddd/adhd/data.html>.

[7] Twenge JM. IGen: why today's super-connected kids are growing up less rebellious, more tolerant, less happy—and completely unprepared for adulthood—and what that means for the rest of us. Simon and Schuster; 2017.

Chapter 17

[1] Martino BD, Kumaran D, Seymour B, Dolan RJ. Frames, biases, and rational decision-making in the human brain. Science. 2006;313(5787):684—7.

[2] Maoz U, Ye S, Ross I, Mamelak A, Koch C. Predicting action content on-line and in real time before action onset — an intracranial human study. In: Pereira F, Burges CJC, Bottou L, Weinberger KQ, editors. Advances in neural information processing systems 25 [Internet]. Curran Associates, Inc.; 2012 [cited 2018 Jun 18]. pp. 872—880. Available from: <http://papers.nips.cc/paper/4513-predicting-action-content-on-line-and-in-real-time-before-action-onset-an-intracranial-human-study.pdf>.

[3] Haynes J-D, Rees G. Neuroimaging: decoding mental states from brain activity in humans. Nat Rev Neurosci 2006;7(7):523—34.

[4] Williams N, Henson RN. Recent advances in functional neuroimaging analysis for cognitive neuroscience. Brain Neurosci Adv 2018;2 :2398212817752727.

[5] Shoham Y. Towards the AI Index. AI Mag 2017;38(4):71—7.

[6] Wehner M. Facebook engineers panic, pull plug on AI after bots develop their own language [Internet]. BGR; 2017 [cited 2018 Jun 1]. Available from: <http://bgr.com/2017/07/31/facebook-ai-shutdown-language/>.

[7] McKay T. No, Facebook did not panic and shut down an AI program that was getting dangerously smart [Internet]. Gizmodo; 2017 [cited 2018 Jun 1]. Available from: <https://gizmodo.com/no-facebook-did-not-panic-and-shut-down-an-ai-program-1797414922>.

[8] Hassabis D, Kumaran D, Summerfield C, Botvinick M. Neuroscience-inspired artificial intelligence. Neuron. 2017;95(2):245—58.

[9] Nedelkoska L, Quintini G. Automation, skills use and training Mar 8; 2018 [cited 2018 Jun 1]. Available from: <https://www.oecd-ilibrary.org/employment/automation-skills-use-and-training_2e2f4eea-en>.

[10] Suárez-Ruiz F, Zhou X, Pham Q-C. Can robots assemble an IKEA chair? Sci Robot 2018;3(17):eaat6385.

[11] Chen N, Ribeiro B, Chen A. Financial credit risk assessment: a recent review. Artif Intell Rev 2016;45(1):1—23.

[12] Amrein-Beardsley A. Breaking news: a big victory in court in houston [Internet]. VAMboozled!; 2017 [cited 2018 Jun 2]. Available from: <http://vamboozled.com/breaking-news-victory-in-court-in-houston/>.

[13] Lee H, Grosse R, Ranganath R, Ng AY. Convolutional deep belief networks for scalable unsupervised learning of hierarchical representations. Proceedings of the 26th annual international conference on machine learning [Internet]. New York, NY, USA: ACM; 2009 [cited 2018 Jun 2]. p. 609−16. (ICML '09).

[14] Goodfellow I, Bengio Y, Courville A. Deep learning. Cambridge, MA: The MIT Press; 2016. p. 775.

[15] Montavon G, Samek W, Müller K-R. Methods for interpreting and understanding deep neural networks. Digit Signal Process 2018;73:1−15.

[16] Jabr F, Jabr F. Know your neurons: how to classify different types of neurons in the brain's forest [Internet]. Scientific American Blog Network; 2012 [cited 2018 Jun 2]. Available from: <https://blogs.scientificamerican.com/brainwaves/know-your-neurons-classifying-the-many-types-of-cells-in-the-neuron-forest/>.

[17] Gold JI, Shadlen MN. The neural basis of decision making. Annu Rev Neurosci 2007;30(1):535−74.

[18] Neumann ID, Landgraf R. Balance of brain oxytocin and vasopressin: implications for anxiety, depression, and social behaviors. Trends Neurosci 2012;35(11):649−59.

[19] Hoogland TM, Parpura V. Editorial: the role of glia in plasticity and behavior. Front Cell Neurosci [Internet]. 2015 [cited 2018 Jun 2]; 9. Available from: <https://www.frontiersin.org/articles/10.3389/fncel.2015.00356/full>.

[20] Luczynski P, McVey Neufeld K-A, Oriach CS, Clarke G, Dinan TG, Cryan JF. Growing up in a bubble: using germ-free animals to assess the influence of the gut microbiota on brain and behavior. Int J Neuropsychopharmacol 2016;19(8) Aug 1 [cited 2018 Jun 2]. Available from: <https://academic.oup.com/ijnp/article/19/8/pyw020/2910071>.

[21] Bryson JJ, Diamantis ME, Grant TD. Of, for, and by the people: the legal lacuna of synthetic persons. Artif Intell Law 2017;25(3):273−91.

Chapter 18

[1] Hurley D. Jumper cables for the mind. The New York Times. November 1, 2013.

[2] Batuman E. Electrified: adventures in transcranial direct-current stimulation. The New Yorker. April 6, 2015.

[3] Oberhaus D. The science and snake oil of neuro stimulation. VICE Motherboard. March 13, 2016.

[4] ABC Radio. Does brain stimulation work? ABC Morning Drive (Melbourne); October 8, 2014.

[5] NOVA Magnetic Mind Control. NOVA: Science Now February 2, 2011.

[6] Horvath JC, Forte JD, Carter O. Quantitative review finds no evidence of cognitive effects in healthy populations from single-session transcranial direct current stimulation (tDCS). Brain Stimul Basic TransClin Res Neuromodul 2015;8(3):535−50.

[7] Horvath JC, Forte JD, Carter O. Evidence that transcranial direct current stimulation (tDCS) generates little-to-no reliable neurophysiologic effect beyond MEP amplitude modulation in healthy human subjects: a systematic review. Neuropsychologia 2015;66:213−36.

[8] Horvath JC, Carter O, Forte JD. Transcranial direct current stimulation: five important issues we aren't discussing (but probably should be). Front Syst Neurosci 2014;8:2.

[9]   Pascual-Leone A, Horvath JC, Robertson EM. Enhancement of normal cognitive abilities through noninvasive brain stimulation. InCortical Connectivity. Berlin Heidelberg: Springer; 2012. p. 207−49.

[10] Westwood SJ, Romani C. Transcranial direct current stimulation (tDCS) modulation of picture naming and word reading: a meta-analysis of single session tDCS applied to healthy participants. Neuropsychologia 2017;104:234−49.

[11] Elsner B, Kugler J, Pohl M, Mehrholz J. Direct electrical current to the brain for language impairment after stroke. Cochrane Libr 2015.

[12] Mancuso LE, Ilieva IP, Hamilton RH, Farah MJ. Does transcranial direct current stimulation improve healthy working memory?: a meta-analytic review. J Cogn Neurosci 2016;28(8):1063−89.

[13] Medina J, Cason S. No evidential value in samples of transcranial direct current stimulation (tDCS) studies of cognition and working memory in healthy populations. Cortex 2017;94:131−41.

[14] Horvath JC, Carter O, Forte JD. No significant effect of transcranial direct current stimulation (tDCS) found on simple motor reaction time comparing 15 different simulation protocols. Neuropsychologia 2016;91:544−52.

[15] Underwood E. Cadaver study challenges brain stimulation methods. Science 2016;352 (6284):397.

[16] Horvath JC, Vogrin SJ, Carter O, Cook MJ, Forte JD. Effects of a common transcranial direct current stimulation (tDCS) protocol on motor evoked potentials found to be highly variable within individuals over 9 testing sessions. Exp Brain Res 2016;234 (9):2629−42.

[17] Chew T, Ho KA, Loo CK. Inter-and intra-individual variability in response to transcranial direct current stimulation (tDCS) at varying current intensities. Brain Stimul Basic Trans Clin Res Neuromodul 2015;8(6):1130−7.

[18] Wörsching J, Padberg F, Helbich K, Hasan A, Koch L, Goerigk S, et al. Test-retest reliability of prefrontal transcranial direct current stimulation (tDCS) effects on functional MRI connectivity in healthy subjects. Neuroimage 2017;155:187−201.

[19] Dyke K, Kim S, Jackson GM, Jackson SR. Intra-subject consistency and reliability of response following 2 mA transcranial direct current stimulation. Brain Stimul Basic Trans Clin Res Neuromodul 2016;9(6):819−25.

[20] Horvath JC, Lodge JM, Hattie J, editors. From the laboratory to the classroom: Translating science of learning for teachers. Routledge; 2016.

Chapter 19

[1]   Thibault RT, Lifshitz M, Birbaumer N, Raz A. Neurofeedback, self-regulation, and brain imaging: clinical science and fad in the service of mental disorders. Psychother Psychosom 2015;84(4):193−207.

[2]   Schönenberg M, Wiedemann E, Schneidt A, et al. Neurofeedback, sham neurofeedback, and cognitive-behavioural group therapy in adults with attention-deficit hyperactivity disorder: a triple-blind, randomised, controlled trial. Lancet Psychiatry 2017;4:673−84.

[3]   Thibault RT, Raz A. The psychology of neurofeedback: clinical intervention even if applied placebo. Am Psychol 2017;72(7):679−88.

[4] Ghaziri J, Tucholka A, Larue V, Blanchette-Sylvestre M, Reyburn G, Gilbert G, et al. Neurofeedback training induces changes in white and gray matter. Clin EEG Neurosci 2013;44(4):265−72.

[5] Macnamara BN, Hambrick DZ, Oswald FL. Deliberate practice and performance in music, games, sports, education, and professions: a meta-analysis. Psychol Sci 2014;25 (8):1608−18.

[6] Watanabe T, Sasaki Y, Shibata K, Kawato M. Advances in fMRI real-time neurofeedback. Trends Cogn Sci 2017;21(12):997−1010.

Chapter 20

[1] SharpBrains. In: SharpBrains: tracking health and wellness applications of brain science; 2014.

[2] Federal Trade Commission. In: Company claimed program would sharpen performance in everyday life and protect against cognitive decline; 2016.

[3] Glickstein M. Golgi and cajal: the neuron doctrine and the 100th anniversary of the 1906 Nobel Prize. Curr Biol 2006;16:R147−51.

[4] Rueda MR, Rothbart MK, McCandliss BD, Saccomanno L, Posner MI. Training, maturation, and genetic influences on the development of executive attention. Proc Natl Acad Sci USA 2005;102:14931−6.

[5] Klingberg T, et al. Computerized training of working memory in children with ADHD—a randomized, controlled trial. J Am Acad Child Adoles Psychiatry 2005;44:177−86.

[6] Ball K, et al. Effects of cognitive training interventions with older adults. JAMA 2002;288:2271−81.

[7] Barnett WS, et al. Educational effects of the tools of the mind curriculum: a randomized trial. Early Childhood Res Q 2008;23:299−313.

[8] Merzenich MM, et al. Temporal processing deficits of language-learning impaired children ameliorated by training. Science 1996;271:77−81.

[9] Diamond A. Activities and programs that improve children's executive functions. Curr Dir Psychol Sci 2012;21:335−41.

[10] Chapman SB, et al. Neural mechanisms of brain plasticity with complex cognitive training in healthy seniors. Cereb Cortex 2013.

[11] Green CS, Bavelier D. Exercising your brain: a review of human brain plasticity and training-induced learning. Psychol Aging 2008;23:692−701.

[12] Tang YY, et al. Short-term meditation induces white matter changes in the anterior cingulate. Proc Natl Acad Sci USA 2010;107:15649−52.

[13] CognitiveTrainingData.org. Cognitive Training Data Response Letter. <https://www.cognitivetrainingdata.org/the-controversy-does-brain-training-work/response-letter/>.

[14] A Consensus on the Brain Training Industry from the Scientific Community, Max Planck Institute for Human Development and Stanford Center on Longevity, accessed Nov 5, 2018, http://longevity3.stanford.edu/blog/2014/10/15/the-consensus-on-the-brain-training-industry-from-the-scientific-community/.

Chapter 21

[1] Purser RE, Forbes D, Burke A, editors. Handbook of mindfulness: culture, context, and social engagement. Springer International Publishing; 2016.
[2] Van Dam NT, van Vugt MK, Vago DR, Schmalzl L, Saron CD, Olendzki A, et al. Mind the hype: a critical evaluation and prescriptive agenda for research on mindfulness and meditation. Perspect Psychol Sci 2018;13(1):36–61.
[3] Congleton C, Hölzel BK, Lazar SW. Mindfulness can literally change your brain. Harvard Bus Rev 2015;309–18.
[4] Begley S. Train your mind, change your brain: how a new science reveals our extraordinary potential to transform ourselves. Random House; 2007.
[5] Thompson E. Meditation, Buddhism, and science. Looping effects and the cognitive science of mindfulness meditation. New York: Oxford University Press; 2017. p. 47–61. Chapter 3.
[6] Fox KC, Nijeboer S, Dixon ML, Floman JL, Ellamil M, Rumak SP, et al. Is meditation associated with altered brain structure? A systematic review and meta-analysis of morphometric neuroimaging in meditation practitioners. Neurosci Biobehav R. 2014;43:48–73.
[7] Tang YY, Hölzel BK, Posner MI. The neuroscience of mindfulness meditation. Nat Rev Neurosci 2015;16(4):213.
[8] Weible AP, Piscopo DM, Rothbart MK, Posner MI, Niell CM. Rhythmic brain stimulation reduces anxiety-related behavior in a mouse model based on meditation training. Proc Natl Acad Sci USA 2017;114(10):2532–7.
[9] Button KS, Ioannidis JP, Mokrysz C, Nosek BA, Flint J, Robinson ES, et al. Power failure: why small sample size undermines the reliability of neuroscience. Nat Rev Neurosci 2013;14(5):365.
[10] Munafò MR, Nosek BA, Bishop DV, Button KS, Chambers CD, du Sert NP, et al. A manifesto for reproducible science. Nat Hum Behav 2017;1:0021.
[11] Fox KC, Dixon ML, Nijeboer S, Girn M, Floman JL, Lifshitz M, et al. Functional neuroanatomy of meditation: a review and meta-analysis of 78 functional neuroimaging investigations. Neurosci Biobehav Res 2016;65:208–28.
[12] Eickhoff SB, Laird AR, Fox PM, Lancaster JL, Fox PT. Implementation errors in the GingerALE Software: description and recommendations. Hum Brain Mapp 2017;38 (1):7–11.
[13] Poldrack RA, Baker CI, Durnez J, Gorgolewski KJ, Matthews PM, Munafò MR, et al. Scanning the horizon: towards transparent and reproducible neuroimaging research. Nat Rev Neurosci 2017;18(2):115–26.
[14] Choudhury S, Slaby J. Critical neuroscience: a handbook of the social and cultural contexts of neuroscience. John Wiley & Sons; 2012.
[15] McMahan DL. Meditation, Buddhism, and science. How meditation works: theorizing the role of cultural context in Buddhist contemplative practices. New York: Oxford University Press; 2017. p. 21–46. Chapter 2.
[16] Kirmayer LJ. Mindfulness in cultural context. Transcult Psychiatry 2015;52 (4):447–69.
[17] Prätzlich M, Kossowsky J, Gaab J, Krummenacher P. Impact of short-term meditation and expectation on executive brain functions. Behav Brain Res 2016;297:268–76.

[18] Farb NA. Mind your expectations: exploring the roles of suggestion and intention in mindfulness training. J Mind-Body Regul 2012;2(1):27−42.

[19] Moerman DE, Jonas WB. Deconstructing the placebo effect and finding the meaning response. Ann Intern Med 2002;136(6):471−6.

[20] Khoury B. Mindfulness: embodied and embedded. Mindfulness 2017;1−6.

[21] Khoury B, Knäuper B, Pagnini F, Trent N, Chiesa A, Carrière K. Embodied mindfulness. Mindfulness 2017;8(5):1160−71.

[22] Johnson W. The posture of meditation: a practical manual for meditators of all traditions. Shambhala Publications; 1996.

[23] Lifshitz M, Thibault RT, Roth RR, Raz A. Source localization of brain states associated with canonical neuroimaging postures. J Cognitive Neurosci 2017;29(7):1292−301.

Chapter 22

[1]   Tucker N. Daniel Amen is the most popular psychiatrist in America. To most researchers and scientists, that's a very bad thing. The Washington Post; 2012.

[2]   Burton R. Brain scam. Salon 2018.

[3]   Choudhury S, Slaby J. Critical neuroscience: a handbook of the social and cultural contexts of neuroscience; 2011.

[4]   Bennett C, Miller M, Wolford G. Neural correlates of interspecies perspective taking in the post-mortem Atlantic Salmon: an argument for multiple comparisons correction. Neuroimage 2009.

[5]   Ali SS, Lifshitz M, Raz A. Empirical neuroenchantment: from reading minds to thinking critically. Front Hum Neurosci 2014.

[6]   Lewandowsky S, Ecker UKH, Seifert CM, Schwarz N, Cook J. Misinformation and its correction: continued influence and successful debiasing. Psychol Sci Public Interes Suppl 2012.

[7]   Lumosity to pay $2 million to settle FTC deceptive advertising charges for its "brain training" program. Federal Trade Commission; 2016.

[8]   Brain Training: Mind Games. Marketplace, CBC; 2015.

[9]   Owen AM, Hampshire A, Grahn JA, Stenton R, Dajani S, Burns AS, et al. Putting brain training to the test. Nature 2010.

[10] Raz A, Rabipour S. How (not) to train your brain. Oxford University Press; 2019.

Chapter 23

[1]   Sporns O. Discovering the human connectome. Cambridge, MA: MIT Press; 2012. xii, 232 pp.

[2]   Sporns O, Tononi G, Kotter R. The human connectome: a structural description of the human brain. PLoS Comput Biol 2005;1(4):e42.

[3]   Bassett DS, Sporns O. Network neuroscience. Nat Neurosci 2017;20(3):353−64.

[4]   Raichle ME. The restless brain: how intrinsic activity organizes brain function. Philos Trans R Soc Lond B Biol Sci 2015;370.

[5]   Logothetis NK. What we can do and what we cannot do with fMRI. Nature 2008;453 (7197):869−78.

[6] Biswal B, Yetkin FZ, Haughton VM, Hyde JS. Functional connectivity in the motor cortex of resting human brain using echo-planar MRI. Magn Reson Med 1995;34 (4):537−41.

[7] Raichle ME, MacLeod AM, Snyder AZ, Powers WJ, Gusnard DA, Shulman GL. A default mode of brain function. Proc Natl Acad Sci USA 2001;98(2):676−82.

[8] Greicius MD, Krasnow B, Reiss AL, Menon V. Functional connectivity in the resting brain: a network analysis of the default mode hypothesis. Proc Natl Acad Sci USA 2003;100(1):253−8.

[9] Smith SM, Fox PT, Miller KL, Glahn DC, Fox PM, Mackay CE, et al. Correspondence of the brain's functional architecture during activation and rest. Proc Natl Acad Sci USA 2009;106(31):13040−5.

[10] Tavor I, Parker Jones O, Mars RB, Smith SM, Behrens TE, Jbabdi S. Task-free MRI predicts individual differences in brain activity during task performance. Science 2016;352(6282):216−20.

[11] Haueis P. Meeting the brain on its own terms. Front Hum Neurosci 2014;8:815.

[12] Van Essen DC, Smith SM, Barch DM, Behrens TE, Yacoub E, Ugurbil K, et al. The WU-Minn human connectome project: an overview. Neuroimage 2013;80:62−79.

[13] Glasser MF, Coalson TS, Robinson EC, Hacker CD, Harwell J, Yacoub E, et al. A multi-modal parcellation of human cerebral cortex. Nature 2016;536(7615):171−8.

[14] Biswal BB, Mennes M, Zuo XN, Gohel S, Kelly C, Smith SM, et al. Toward discovery science of human brain function. Proc Natl Acad Sci USA 2010;107(10):4734−9.

[15] Haueis P. Meeting the brain on its own terms. Exploratory concept formation and non-cognitive functions in neuroscience: Otto-von-Guericke Universitaet; 2017.

Chapter 24

[1] Uttal WR. The new phrenology: the limits of localizing cognitive processes in the brain. Cambridge: MIT Press; 2001.

[2] Hubbard EM. A discussion and review of Uttal (2001) The New Phrenology. Cogn Sci Online 2003;1:22−33.

[3] Hohwy J. Functional integration and the mind. Synthese 2007;159:315−28.

[4] Eickhoff SB, Constable RT, Yeo BTT. Topographic organization of the cerebral cortex and brain cartography. Neuroimage 2018;170:332−47.

[5] Deco G, Kringelbach ML. Great expectations: using whole-brain computational connectomics for understanding neuropsychiatric disorders. Neuron 2014;84:892−905.

[6] Deco G, Cabral J, Woolrich M, Stevner ABA, Van Hartevelt T, Kringelbach ML. Single or multi-frequency generators in on-going MEG data: a mechanistic whole-brain model of empirical MEG data. Neuroimage 2017;152:538−50.

[7] Deco G, Jirsa V, McIntosh AR, Sporns O, Kotter R. Key role of coupling, delay, and noise in resting brain fluctuations. Proc Natl Acad Sci USA 2009;106(25):10302−7.

[8] Deco G, Jirsa VK, McIntosh AR. Emerging concepts for the dynamical organization of resting state activity in the brain. Nat Rev Neurosci 2011;12:43−56.

[9] Kringelbach ML, McIntosh AR, Ritter P, Jirsa VK, Deco G. The rediscovery of slowness: exploring the timing of cognition. TICS 2015;19(10):616−28.

[10] Cabral J, Kringelbach ML, Deco G. Functional connectivity dynamically evolves on multiple time-scales over a static structural connectome: models and mechanisms. Neuroimage 2017;160:84−96.

[11] Atasoy S, Donnelly I, Pearson J. Human brain networks function in connectome-specific harmonic waves. Nat Commun 2016;7.

[12] Raichle ME, Snyder AZ. A default mode of brain function: a brief history of an evolving idea. Neuroimage 2007;37(4):1083−90 discussion 1097−9.

[13] Biswal B, Yetkin FZ, Haughton VM, Hyde JS. Functional connectivity in the motor cortex of resting human brain using echo-planar MRI. Magn Reson Med 1995;34 (4):537−41.

[14] Deco G, Kringelbach ML. Metastability and coherence: extending the communication through coherence hypothesis using a whole-brain computational perspective. Trends Neurosci 2016;39(3):125−35.

[15] Deco G, Tononi G, Boly M, Kringelbach ML. Rethinking segregation and integration: contributions of whole-brain modelling. Nat Rev Neurosci 2015;16:430−9.

[16] Deco G, McIntosh AR, Shen K, Hutchison RM, Menon RS, Everling S, et al. Identification of optimal structural connectivity using functional connectivity and neural modeling. J Neurosci 2014;34(23):7910−16.

[17] Ghosh A, Rho Y, McIntosh AR, Kotter R, Jirsa VK. Noise during rest enables the exploration of the brain's dynamic repertoire. PLoS Comput Biol 2008;4(10): e1000196.

[18] Jirsa VK, Jantzen KJ, Fuchs A, Kelso JAS. Spatiotemporal forward solution of the EEG and MEG using network modeling. Med Imaging, IEEE Trans 2002;21 (5):493−504.

[19] Johansen-Berg H, Rushworth MF. Using diffusion imaging to study human connectional anatomy. Annu Rev Neurosci 2009;32:75−94.

[20] Berridge KC, Kringelbach ML. Pleasure systems in the brain. Neuron 2015;86:646−64.

[21] Kringelbach ML, Phillips H. Emotion: pleasure and pain in the brain. Oxford: Oxford University Press; 2014.

[22] Atasoy S, Deco G, Kringelbach ML, Pearson J. Harmonic brain modes: a unifying framework for linking space and time in brain dynamics. Neuroscientist 2018;24:277−93.

[23] Deco G, Van Hartevelt T, Fernandes HM, Stevner ABA, Kringelbach ML. The most relevant human brain regions for functional connectivity: evidence for a dynamical workspace of binding nodes from whole-brain computational modelling. Neuroimage 2017;146:197−210.

[24] Biswal BB, Mennes M, Zuo XN, Gohel S, Kelly C, Smith SM, et al. Toward discovery science of human brain function. Proc Natl Acad Sci USA 2010;107(10):4734−9.

[25] Kringelbach ML, Green AL, Aziz TZ. Balancing the brain: resting state networks and deep brain stimulation. Front Integr Neurosci 2011;5:8.

[26] Kahan J, Papadaki A, White M, Mancini L, Yousry T, Zrinzo L, et al. The safety of using body-transmit MRI in patients with implanted deep brain stimulation devices. PLoS One 2015;10(6):e0129077.

[27] Saenger VM, Kahan J, Foltynie T, Friston K, Aziz TZ, Green AL, et al. Uncovering the underlying mechanisms and whole-brain dynamics of therapeutic deep brain stimulation for Parkinson's disease [bioRxiv 083162]. Sci Rep 2017;7(1):9882.

[28] Carhart-Harris RL, Bolstridge M, Rucker J, Day CMJ, Erritzoe D, Kaelen M, et al. Psilocybin with psychological support for treatment-resistant depression: an open-label feasibility study. Lancet Psychiatry 2016;3(7):619−27.

[29] Deco G, Cruzat J, Cabral J, Knudsen GM, Carhart-Harris RL, Whybrow PC, et al. Whole-brain multimodal neuroimaging model links human anatomy, function and neuromodulation: serotonin receptor maps explain non-linear functional effects of LSD. Curr Biol 2018; in press.

Chapter 25

[1] Petersen SE, Posner MI. The attention system of the human brain: 20 years after. Annu Rev Neurosci 2012;35:71−89.

[2] Crottaz-Herbtte S, Menon V. Where and when the anterior cingulate cortex modulate-sattentional response: combined fMRI and ERP evidence. J Cogn Neurosci 2006;18:766−80.

[3] Kosslyn SM. Image and brain: the resolution of the imagery debate. Cambridge MA: MIT Press; 1994.

[4] Ochsner KN, Bunge SA, Gross JJ, Gabrieli JDE. Rethinking feelings: an fMRI study of the cognitive regulation of emotion. J Cogn Neurosci 2002;14:1215−29.

[5] Beauregard M, Levesque J, Bourgouin P. Neural correlates of conscious self-regulation of emotion. J Neurosci 2001;21(RC165):1−6.

[6] Posner MI, Raichle ME. Images of mind. Scientific American Books; 1994.

[7] Rothbart MK, Rueda MR. The development of effortful control. In: Mayr U, Awh E, Keele SW, editors. Developing individuality in the human brain: a tribute to Michael I. Posner. Washington, DC: American Psychological Association; 2005. p. 167−88.

[8] Moffitt TE, Arseneault L, Belsky D, Dickson N, Hancox RJ, Harrington HL, et al. A gradient of childhood self-control predicts health, wealth and public safety. Proc Natl Acad Sci USA 2011;108(7):2693−8.

[9] Posner MI, Tang YY, Lynch G. Mechanisms of white matter change induced by meditation. Front Psychol 2014.

[10] Deisseroth K, Feng G, Majewska AK, Miesenbock G, Ting A, Schnitzer MJ. Next-generation optical technologies for illuminating genetically targeted brain circuits. J Neurosci 2006;26(41):10380−6.

[11] Piscopo DM, Weible AP, Rothbart MK, Posner MI, Niell CM. Changes in white matter resulting form low-frequency brain stimulation. Proc Natl Acad Sci USA 2018;115/27: E6339−46.

[12] Fair DA, Dosenbach NUF, Church JA, Cohen AL, Brahmbhatt S, Miezin FM, et al. Development of distinct control networks through segregation and integration. Proc Natl Acad Sci USA 2007;104(33):13507−12.

[13] Mitra A, Kraft A, Wright P, Acland B, Snyder AZ, Roenthal Z, et al. Spontaenous infra-slow brain activity has unique spatiotemporal dynamis can laminsr structure. Neuron 2018;98:1.

Chapter 26

[1] Damadian R, Goldsmith M, Minkoff L. NMR in cancer: XVI. FONAR image of the live human body. Physiol Chem Phys 1977;9(1):97−100.

[2] Purcell E, Torrey H, Pound R. Resonance absorption by nuclear magnetic moments in a solid. Phys Rev 1946;69:37.

[3] Bloch F. Nuclear induction. Phys Rev 1946;70:460−74.

[4] Chen CN, Sank VJ, Cohen SM, Hoult DI. The field dependence of NMR imaging. I. Laboratory assessment of signal-to-noise ratio and power deposition. Magn Reson Med 1986;3:722−9.

[5] Robitaille PM, Abduljalil AM, Kangarlu A, Zhang X, Yu Y, Burgess R, et al. Human magnetic resonance imaging at 8 T. NMR Biomed 1998;11(6):263−5.

[6]   Kangarlu A, Abduljalil AM, Schwarzbauer C, Norris DG, Robitaille PM. Human rapid acquisition with relaxation enhancement imaging at 8 T without specific absorption rate violation. MAGMA 1999;9(1-2):81−4.

[7]   Kangarlu A, Baertlein BA, Lee R, Ibrahim T, Yang L, Abduljalil AM, et al. Dielectric resonance phenomena in ultra high field MRI. J Comput Assist Tomogr 1999;23 (6):821−31.

[8]   Kangarlu A, Burgess RE, Zhu H, Nakayama T, Hamlin RL, Abduljalil AM, et al. Cognitive, cardiac, and physiological safety studies in ultra high field magnetic resonance imaging. Magn Reson Imaging 1999;17(10):1407−16.

[9]   Ogawa S, Lee TM, Kay AR, Tank DW. Brain magnetic resonance imaging with contrast dependent on blood oxygenation. Proc Natl Acad Sci USA 1990;87(24):9868−72.

[10] Tkác I, Oz G, Adriany G, Uğurbil K, Gruetter R. In vivo 1H NMR spectroscopy of the human brain at high magnetic fields: metabolite quantification at 4T vs. 7T. Magn Reson Med 2009;62(4):868−79.

[11] LeBihan D. IVIM method measures diffusion and perfusion. Diagn Imaging (San Franc). 1990;12(6):133−6.

[12] Hyde JS, Li R. Functional connectivity in rat brain at 200 μm resolution. Brain Connect 2014;4(7):470−80.

[13] Chaimow D, Uğurbil K, Shmuel A. Optimization of functional MRI for detection, decoding and high-resolution imaging of the response patterns of cortical columns. Neuroimage 2018;164:67−99.

[14] Stucht D, Danishad KA, Schulze P, Godenschweger F, Zaitsev M, Speck O. Highest resolution in vivo human brain MRI using prospective motion correction. PLoS One 2015;10(7):e0133921.

[15] Heidemann RM, Ivanov D, Trampel R, Fasano F, Meyer H, Pfeuffer J, et al. Isotropic submillimeter fMRI in the human brain at 7 T: combining reduced field-of-view imaging and partially parallel acquisitions. Magn Reson Med 2012;68(5):1506−16.

[16] Uludağ K, Müller-Bierl B, Uğurbil K. An integrative model for neuronal activity-induced signal changes for gradient and spin echo functional imaging. Neuroimage 2009;48(1):150−65.

[17] Ibrahim TS, Lee R, Baertlein BA, Kangarlu A, Robitaille PL. Application of finite difference time domain method for the design of birdcage RF head coils using multi-port excitations. Magn Reson Imaging 2000;18(6):733−42.

[18] Setsompop K, Cohen-Adad J, Gagoski BA, Raij T, Yendiki A, Keil B, et al. Improving diffusion MRI using simultaneous multi-slice echo planar imaging. Neuroimage 2012;63(1):569−80.

[19] Lewis LD, Setsompop K, Rosen BR, Polimeni JR. Fast fMRI can detect oscillatory neural activity in humans. Proc Natl Acad Sci USA 2016;113(43):E6679−85.

[20] Ibrahim TS, Lee R, Baertlein BA, Kangarlu A, Robitaille PL. Application of finite difference time domain method for the design of birdcage RF head coils using multi-port excitations. Magn Reson Imaging 2000;18(6):733−42.

[21] Poser BA, Anderson RJ, Guérin B, Setsompop K, Deng W, Mareyam A, et al. Simultaneous multislice excitation by parallel transmission. Magn Reson Med 2014;71 (4):1416−27.

[22] Pohmann R, Speck O, Scheffler K. Signal-to-noise ratio and MR tissue parameters in human brain imaging at 3, 7, and 9.4 tesla using current receive coil arrays. Magn Reson Med 2016;75:801−9.

[23] Chung JJ, Choi W, Jin T, Lee JH, Kim S-G. Chemical-exchange-sensitive MRI of amide, amine and NOE at 9.4 T versus 15.2 T. NMR Biomed 2017;30:e3740.

[24] Mlynárik V, Cudalbu C, Xin L, Gruetter R. 1H NMR spectroscopy of rat brain in vivo at 14.1Tesla: improvements in quantification of the neurochemical profile. J Magn Reson 2008;194:163—8.
[25] New insights into brain function with molecular and functional MRI of the rodent brain at ultra-high fields|Bruker: <https://www.bruker.com/service/education-training/webinars/pci-webinars/new-insights-into-brain-function-with-molecular-and-functional-mri-of-the-rodent-brain-at-ultra-high-fields.html>.

Chapter 27

[1] Swanson LW, Newman E, Araque A, Dubinsky JM. The beautiful brain: the drawings of Santiago Ramón y Cajal. New York: Abrams; 2017.
[2] Margulies DS, Böttger J, Watanabe A, Gorgolewski KJ. Visualizing the human connectome. NeuroImage 2013;80:445—61.
[3] Seligman R, Choudhury S, Kirmayer LJ. Locating culture in the brain and in the world: from social categories to the ecology of mind. In: Chiao J, editor. The Oxford handbook of cultural neuroscience. Oxford: Oxford University Press; 2015.
[4] Han S, Northoff G, Vogeley K, Wexler BE, Kitayama S, Varnum ME. A cultural neuroscience approach to the biosocial nature of the human brain. Ann Rev Psychol 2013;64:335—59.
[5] Konvalinka I, Roepstorff A. The two-brain approach: how can mutually interacting brains teach us something about social interaction? Front Hum Neurosci 2012;6:215.
[6] Molenberghs P. The neuroscience of in-group bias. Neurosci Biobehav Rev 2013;37(8):1530—6.
[7] Heyes C. Cognitive gadgets: the cultural evolution of thinking. Harvard University Press; 2018.
[8] Ramstead MJ, Veissière SP, Kirmayer LJ. Cultural affordances: scaffolding local worlds through shared intentionality and regimes of attention. Front Psychol 2016;7.
[9] Veissiere S. Thinking through other minds: a variational approach to cognition and culture. (Submitted).
[10] Gibbs Jr RW. Embodiment and cognitive science. Cambridge University Press; 2005.
[11] Gallagher S. Enactivist interventions: rethinking the mind. Oxford University Press; 2017.
[12] Dehaene S. Reading in the brain: the new science of how we read. Penguin; 2009.

Index

Printed in the United States
By Bookmasters